THE BLACK AGED
IN THE UNITED STATES

THE BLACK AGED
IN THE UNITED STATES
An Annotated Bibliography

LENWOOD G. DAVIS

GREENWOOD PRESS
WESTPORT, CONNECTICUT • LONDON, ENGLAND

Library of Congress Cataloging in Publication Data

Davis, Lenwood G
  The Black aged in the United States.

  Includes index.
  1. Afro-American aged—Bibliography. 2. Old age
assistance—United States—Bibliography. I. Title.
Z7164.04D38 [HQ1064.U6]   016.3052'6'08996073
ISBN 0-313-22560-5 (lib. bdg.)   80-1193

Library of Congress Catalog Card Number: 80-1193
ISBN: 0-313-22560-5

First published in 1980

Greenwood Press
A division of Congressional Information Service, Inc.
88 Post Road West, Westport, Connecticut 06881

Printed in the United States of America

10 9 8 7 6 5 4 3 2 1

To
Beaulah A. Pickett,
an ageless Black Woman

Contents

Foreword

Although our techniques for prolonging life have improved, our tolerance for the handicaps confronting the aged seems to have declined. We need to flex our political muscle a little more in demanding a fair shake for this neglected minority from our society. This book dramatizes the plight of older people in this country, and it also points to hopeful signs that more scholarly research on the aged will herald significant change.

More than three hundred years ago, William Shakespeare wrote, "Crabbed age and youth cannot live together. Youth is full of pleasance, age is full of care." It is difficult to overstate the cares of age, among them loneliness, economic insecurity, anxiety about health, disappointment with children, inability to keep creatively involved in society's affairs, and generally, psychological "hangups" about aging. Problems are compounded for Blacks who have suffered a lifetime of indignities and injustices.

The 1970 census shows that Black people comprise 8 percent of the 20 million people who are over 65. The life expectancy for White men remains the same at 67.5; however, for Black men it has gone down since the 1960s, from 61.1 years to 60.0. Life expectancy for White women rose to 74.9, but only to 67.5 for the Black female.

The economic difference between Whites and Blacks is amazing. The income of aged Blacks runs about half that of Whites. By one estimate, about 90 percent of the aged Black females who are single live in poverty (Gerald Leinward, ed., *Growing Old* [New York, 1975], pp. 9, 35, 46).

According to a recent report by Aaron Henry, a member of the Board of Directors of the National Center on Black Aged in Washington, many aged Blacks who worked in low paying jobs and who originally were excluded from social security must continue to work to feed and clothe themselves, even though they should have retired years ago. At a Philadelphia conference on the Black aged, Henry stated that "jobs such as house maids, chauffeurs and cotton pickers—the only types of jobs the majority of Black people could find, because racism prevented them from getting other types of work—were not covered by the Social Security Act.''

Because the average Black man's life expectancy is well below age 65, he will never be able to collect social security even if he has had work that provided for this. The average Black woman, if she has contributed, will have social security for only 2.5 years (Richard D. Davis, ed., *Aging: Prospects and Issues* [Los Angeles, California, 1973], p. 108).

Over the past few years, there has been a tremendous amount of attention given to the study of "old folks" in this society, which is essential since there are about 21 million people over the age of 65 in the United States today—about 11 percent of the total population. But not enough attention has been paid to the Black aged, and certainly not enough studies focus on aged slaves. Although writers and scholars such as Kenneth M. Stampp, Earl E. Thorpe, Margaret Cartwright, Angela Davis, Eugene D. Genovese, John Brown, Mercer Langston, Charles Ball, Solomon Northrup, Frederick Douglass, Harriet Tubman, Louis Hughes, Austin Steward, William Wells Brown, and George P. Rawick have included some commentary on the Black aged slave in their writings, there is a limited number of monographs on the subject. Thus, a bibliography on this subject can fill an important niche for anyone seeking to locate dependable references on the subject.

Many scholars have written bibliographies on various aspects of American history, but none has compiled as many bibliographies on Black history as has Lenwood Davis. His eighty bibliographies are valuable tools for scholars who wish to examine the historical experiences of Afro-Americans. In this work, the most distinctive aspect of Davis' research is his uncovering of sources on aged slaves—the "griots" of the plantation.

Users of this bibliography must realize that an aged slave "in those days" would have been in her/his thirties. Even today, in some societies, persons are considered to be aged at forty, although sixty-five is the determining age in the developed nations. Dr. Davis chooses to impose the more contemporary numerical category for determining which slaves are aged, that is, those in their sixties.

This bibliography presents annotations of articles, books, dissertations, and theses concerned with various aspects of the Black aged. Therefore, it serves as a reference book for those who wish to learn more about the lives, achievements, and shortcomings of Black aged people. This group is not usually acknowledged by gerontologists as possessing unique problems of color and gender. That the people herein investigated are poorer than their white counterparts amply vindicates this study as a worthwhile venture in gerontological studies.

This new book, then, which pulls together a vast amount of literature on this group, contains a superior collection of sources on the subject, all of which contribute toward supplying a research instrument in the fields of gerontology, Black studies, anthropology, Black history, American history, sociology, psychology, and social work.

The Older Americans Act of 1965, amended in 1976, declares that "older people of our nation are entitled to . . . immediate benefit from proven research knowledge which can sustain and improve health and happiness. . . ." Professor Davis' collection will certainly aid in the realization of that goal, in particular as it applies to the Black aged community.

Dr. Gossie Harold Hudson
Department of History
Morgan State University
Baltimore, Maryland

Introduction

Currently there is a tremendous interest in the United States in its aged. The Black aged have been neglected as a group, since most gerontologists do not acknowledge their problems as any different from those of the White aged. That contention has been challenged by writers such as Jacquelyne J. Jackson, James H. Carter, Gossie H. Hudson, Bonnie J. Gillespie, and others. They believe that the Black aged have special and different problems, since they are for the most part poorer than their white counterparts. For the elderly Black female it is even worse. She is not in "triple jeopardy," she is in "quadruple jeopardy"—Black, old, poor, and female.

Blacks themselves have always taken care of their senior citizens, since long before they came to the United States. In African society elders were the leaders and most respected members of the community. Even during slavery in America during the 1800s the Black elderly were looked upon with respect by both slaves and free Blacks. Moreover, free Blacks during the slave era founded organizations that had as their primary objective the care for the elderly, widows, and orphans. Blacks have traditionally made special efforts to care for their old, sick, and homeless.

Another little-known fact is that Blacks with the assistance of Whites established homes for the Black aged even during the slave era. One of the earliest homes was the Home For Aged Colored Women that was founded in Boston about 1860. Another was the Stephen Smith Home for the Aged that was organized in 1864 in Philadelphia. Although there were between two and three hundred homes established for the Black aged between 1860 and the present, the Stephen Smith Home is one of the few that is presently still in existence and functioning.

Although presently there is an increased awareness of the plight of the Black elderly, some attention should be focused on the historical role of the Black aged because their role has not changed drastically in some ways since slavery. They still are, in many instances, the stabilizing force in the Black family structure.

While writers such as Herbert G. Gutman, Leslie Howard Owen, Kenneth M. Stampp, Eugene D. Genovese, Robert W. Fogel, Stanley L. Engerman, J. C. Furmas, Bishop Meade, Joseph H. Ingraham, Nehemiah Adams, Stanley Feldstein, Bertram W. Doyle, James Redpath, and others give their impressions of the status of the aged slave, it is the narratives of former slaves such as Frederick Douglass, Solomon Northup, Louis Hughes, Austin Steward, William Wells Brown, Charles Ball, John Brown, John Mercer Langston, and others who give us a clearer picture of the position of the elderly slaves and the way they were treated.

There are two arguments concerning the status of aged slaves presented in these selections. One position is that old slaves were not cared for by their masters but left to beg in the streets for a scanty and precarious subsistence. Old slaves were "doctored up" and sold for less than a good dog, in one case for a mere dollar. Another instance involved a slave who was sold for a meager ten dollars. Still another case shows that two aged slaves were sold together for only thirteen dollars. Some aged slaves were not cared for when they were ill but were left to die. Other accounts state that old slaves were mistreated and even whipped by their mistresses and masters. One writer states that masters emancipated some aged slaves as a reward for a lifetime of faithful service, "but other planters intended many of these seeming generosities simply as part of a larger scheme to set themselves and their relatives free of responsibility for care of the old persons." Although some of the slaves were in their 80s and 90s they still waited on their mistresses and masters. They had to continue to work to "pay" for their support.

The other argument is that old slaves were properly cared for by their masters after years of services. Some writers note that some planters built cottages for old slaves and provided them with "pensions." Other authors add that aged slaves had the "light" duties of babysitters, nurses, seamstresses, cooks, weavers, and coach drivers. Another author contends that "the aged slaves had a high degree of security, emotional as well as physical." "Their master's error," this writer continues, "lay in the supposition that the modest protection of the Big House accounted for their widespread cheerfulness and contentment, for the old folks' ability to live decently and with self-respect depended primarily on the support of their younger fellow slaves."

Some of the slave narratives and slave testimonies state that some old slaves had "light" duties and that some were mistreated. What is most significant, however, is that the narratives and testimonies tell us how the slaves themselves viewed their aged members. Frederick Douglass, for example, recalls the influence that his grandmother had on him during the period that he was a slave. Douglass surmises that his grandmother's kindness and love stood in the place of his mother, whom he did not know. His grandmother, according to Douglass, was a woman of power and spirit.

The abolitionist also argues that the mechanics were called "uncles" by all of the younger slaves, not because they really sustained that relationship to any, but according to plantation etiquette, as a mark of respect due from the younger to older slaves. He concludes that "strange, and even ridiculous as it may seem, among a people so uncultivated, and with so many stern trials to look in the face, there is not to be found, among any people, a more rigid enforcement of the law of respect to elders, than they maintain. . . ."

Solomon Northup, another ex-slave, wrote that aged slaves were patriarchs among other slaves. He recalls "Old Abran was a kindhearted being, a sort of patriarch among us, fond of entertaining his younger brethren with grave and serious discourse. He was deeply versed in such philosophy as is taught in the cabin of the slave." Louis Hughes declares that when a slave woman was too old to do much of anything, she was assigned to be in charge of young babies in the absence of their mothers, usually with no one to help her. Austin Steward, a slave for twenty-two years and a freeman for forty years, recalls how the old slaves were treated on his former plantation in Virginia. According to him, his mistress had old slaves "punished by having them severely whipped by a man, which she never failed to do for every trifling fault."

William Wells Brown states that one of his jobs was to prepare the old slaves for the slave market. He remembers shaving the old men's beards and plucking out their gray hairs. If there were too many gray hairs, he colored them black. The owner passed these slaves off as being middle-aged, thereby cheating the buyers. Brown also mentions an old slave called "Uncle Frank," who was a fortune-teller. He told both slaves' and planters' fortunes. Charles Ball relates that as a child he passed many long nights with his grandfather "listening to his narratives of the scenes through which he had passed in Africa," and hearing of his grandpa's religion with its strong injunction of "tenderness to wives and children."

John Brown, an ex-slave from Georgia, recollects that on his plantation there was an old slave by the name of "Minney," the mother of thirteen children, who was stoned by her master because she would not run fast enough for him. Her master laughed after the stone broke her arm. The author also describes how old "Aunties" and "Uncles" generally took care of the sick, using methods learned from other slaves over the years. John Mercer Langston, a former slave, and the first Black elected from Virginia to the United States House of Representatives, recalls that his master freed his aged slaves in his will. One, Billy Quarles, was also given two hundred and twenty dollars.

Later testimonies of ex-slaves support the positions of the slave narratives concerning the aged slave as explained by many slaves whose stories are told in George P. Rawick's *The American Slave: A Composite Autobiography*. Three ex-slaves from Georgia, Georgia Baker, Martha Colquitt, and Callier

Elder, recall the influence that their grandparents had on them. Georgia Baker declares she spent much of her early childhood in the company of her grandfather, who slept "on a trundle bed in the kitchen" and who tended Georgia and her siblings while their parents were in the fields. Martha Colquitt states her grandmother helped provide material comfort for her: "Grandma helped to cook, wash, and make clothes." Callier Elder recalls that her "Grandpa helped supply wild nuts, garden produce, and meat for the family table." Perry Jemison, a former slave from Ohio, remembers that "My grandmother wuz named Snooky and my grandfather Anthony. I thought der wuzn't a better friend in all de world den my grandmother. She would do all she could for her grandchildren. Der wuz no food allowance for chillun that could not work and my grandmother fed us out of her and my mother's allowance." Austin Grant, of Texas, says that his grandfather used to "tell us things, to keep the whip off our backs."

One of the most interesting stories about aged slaves is discussed in William Still's *The Underground Railroad.* The author writes about Jane Davis, a slave woman of about seventy, from the Eastern Shore section of Maryland. She was a mother of twelve children and "married." Because she was often mistreated and about to be sold to a new master, she decided to leave her children and husband and escape to Buffalo, New York where her brother was living. She escaped by the Underground Railroad. Although she was nearly seventy years old, she slept in the woods for nearly three weeks with little or no food. The author concludes that Miss Davis doubtless represents thousands of aged slave mothers, who, after having been worn out under the yoke, were frequently either offered for sale for a trifle, turned out to die, or compelled to eke out their existence on the most stingy allowance.

Other slaves' testimonies presented here point out that aged slaves were "highly esteemed by both the slaves and the masters." One writer argues that often the aged female slave was the "confidential adviser" of the older members of the slave household. Moreover, the aged slave added "dignity" to her position and "her regime." According to some, the "grannies" were genuine matriarchs—powerful, stabilizing figures who performed a profoundly important service. The slave testimonies reveal that younger slaves learned trades from older slaves. In many instances the "granny" or aged slave was a kind of "gloried nurse and was the authority in nursery matters." The younger slave who attended to the children as guardian and companion, and who was called "nurse," was subordinate to her. Another writer notes that an old slave woman might act as plantation physician, midwife, and, more or less secretly, "witch doctor." One writer gives his idea of the aged slave's role in the "courtship" of slaves on plantations. The author states that almost every large plantation had an experienced old slave who instructed young male slaves in the delicate matter of winning the girls of their choice.

A Northerner who traveled in the South gives an interesting account of his conversation with an old slave. According to the writer, the aged female slave's maternal affection for her children was very strong. The aged slave emphasized that she and other slaves "were not" content to be in slavery contrary to reports of White plantation owners.

Although the foregoing accounts give various roles of and attitudes toward aged slaves, it is noted by Kenneth M. Stampp, Theodore Weld, Robert Fogel, Stanley L. Engerman and others that in 1860 only 1.2 percent of slaves were over seventy; thus the owner of as many as a hundred slaves seldom had more than one or two elderly slaves to support. In many cases a slave was considered "old" at about thirty or thirty-five, and few lived beyond fifty-five. Fogel and Engerman add that "40 percent of the slaves died before age nineteen."

Hence, it can be seen that the aged slave played a vital part on the plantation and was treated with respect by the younger slaves. Perhaps the younger slaves were aware that most of them would not reach old age. What is most important is that aged slaves knew that they had to share their knowledge and experience with younger slaves in the hopes that they would beat the "slave system." Some aged slaves could no longer tolerate the system and escaped to freedom. While other aged slaves were content with their own status, since most knew that they were too old to escape to freedom, they assisted and sometimes encouraged younger slaves to escape, in hopes that they would live their lives in "free" territory and not under the yoke of slavery.

One of the greatest contributions that the aged slaves made to the Black race was that of transmitting the Black culture. The aged slave was usually the closest one to Africa and had more knowledge about it than younger generations. It was she or he who transmitted the history and songs of Africa. One writer points out that one of Black children's chief diversions was to listen to the songs and tales of Africa from their grandparents. Thus the Black aged played a significant role then, as well as now, because they were and are the transmitters of the Black heritage.

There are a number of organizations, institutions, centers, and individuals that have done extensive research on the Black aged since the mid 1970s. The National Center on Black Aged in Washington, D.C., is the leading organization that does research on the Black aged. It puts out a number of studies and reports and also holds various conferences on the Black elderly. The Center for the Study of Aging and Human Development at Duke University Medical School is another leading institution engaged in research on the Black aged. Other institutions such as the Ethel Percy Andrus Gerontology Center at the University of Southern California, the Institute of Gerontology at the University of Michigan-Wayne State University, and the

Center on Aging at San Diego State University have done extensive research on the Black aged. The National Council on the Aging as well as the federal government also put out a number of studies and reports on the Black aged.

The leading individual author on the Black aged is Jacquelyne Johnson Jackson of Duke University Medical School. She has written one book and more than forty articles on the Black aged and edited several books. She has also presented many scholarly papers at major national and international conferences. James H. Carter of Duke University Medical School has also written many articles on the Black aged. The late Hobart H. Jackson, founder of the National Caucus for The Black Aged, wrote a number of articles, as has Gossie H. Hudson of Morgan State University. Others that have written several works are listed in this book. The above, however, deserve special acknowledgment.

Most of the works cited can be located in a good library. The majority of the references in this work can be found at Duke University, University of North Carolina at Chapel Hill, Howard University, Wake Forest University, University of Michigan, Wayne State University, University of Southern California and San Diego State University. Works published by organizations, such as the National Center on Black Aged, and the National Council on The Aging, can be obtained directly from them.

This work could not have been completed without the assistance of many people, to whom I am grateful. I would like to especially thank the following individuals: Janet L. Sims of Howard University for making available to me a number of works located at Howard University; Belinda S. Daniels of Winston-Salem State University for securing many works through interlibrary loan; Sheila Campbell, Felicia Neal and Karen Cox for typing the rough draft of this work; Barbara Laughinghouse for editing and typing the final draft; Jeanett Moore for proofreading this work and giving some valuable suggestions; and last, but not necessarily least, Phyliss Davis, my wife, who tolerated me while working on this project and who has a deep respect for all aged people.

Although this is the most comprehensive annotated bibliography on the Black aged ever compiled, a limited number of books, articles, reports, and other works are excluded because for various reasons they were not available to the compiler. I welcome any additions from readers since I hope to revise this work in the future.

1.

BLACK
AGED AND SLAVERY

Books

Ball, Charles. <u>Slavery in The United States: A Narrative
of the Life and Adventures of Charles Ball, A Black
Man, Who Lived Forty Years in Maryland, South Carolina and Georgia, As A Slave Under Various Masters,
and Was One Year in The Navy With Commodore Barney
During The Late War</u>. Lewiston, Pa.: J. W. Shugert,
1836.

As a child the author recalls that he passed many
long nights with his grandfather "listening to his narrative of the scenes through which he had passed in
Africa," and hearing of his grandpa's religion with
its strong injunctions of "tenderness to wives and
children."

Brown, John. <u>Slave Life in Georgia: A Narrative of the
Life, Sufferings, and Escape of John Brown, A Fugitive
Slave, Now in England</u>. Edited by Louis Alexis Chame-
rovzow. London: Anti-Slavery Society, 1855.

The author points out that old slaves were mistreated.
Brown recalls that an old slave by the name of Mirney,
the mother of thirteen children, was stoned by her master because she would not run fast enough for him.
Her master even laughed at her after the stone broke
her arm. The writer argues that slaves, young and old,
were "doctored" up to look younger when they were being
sold. He also states that old "Aunties" and "Uncles"
generally took care of the sick. They learned this
"trade" from other slaves over the years.

Brown, William Wells. <u>Narrative of William W. Brown, A
Fugitive Slave</u>. Boston: The Anti-Slavery Office,
1847.

The author states that one of his jobs was to prepare

(Brown, William Wells)

the old slaves for the slave market. Mr. Brown was
ordered to shave the old men's beards and pluck out
their gray hairs. If there were too many gray hairs,
he colored them black. After "doctoring" the slaves,
they looked ten or fifteen years younger. The owner
passed those old slaves off as being middle aged;
thereby cheating the buyers, especially in ages of the
slaves which they bought. Mr. Brown also mentions a
slave called "Uncle Frank," who was a fortune teller.
He told slaves and Whites fortunes.

Craft, William and Ellen Craft. Running A Thousand Miles
    For Freedom, Or, The Escape of William and Ellen Craft
    From Slavery.   London: William Tweedie, 1860.

One of the writers, William Craft, points out that although his old master had the reputation of being a
very humane and Christian man, he thought nothing of
selling his aged father and mother, at separate times
to different slave owners. He also argues that his
aged parents were very religious and devoted to the
service of God. The reason his master sold his parents, and other aged slaves, was that "they were getting old, and would soon become valueless in the market, and therefore he intended to sell off all the
old stock, and buy in a young lot."

Douglass, Frederick. My Bondage and My Freedom. New York:
    Miller, Orton and Mulligan, 1855.

The writer states that the mechanics were called "uncles" by all the younger slaves, not because they
really sustained that relationship to any, but according to plantation etiquette, as a mark of respect,
due from the younger to the older slaves. The orator
declares, "strange, and even ridiculous as it may seem,
among a people so uncultivated, and with so many stern
trials to look in the face, there is not to be found,
among any people, a more rigid enforcement of the law
of respect to elders, than they maintain." He continues to say that "a young slave must approach the
company of the older with hat in hand, and woe betide
him, if he fails to acknowledge a favor, of any sort,
with the accustomed 'tank'ee,' etc. So uniformly are
good manners enforced among slaves, that I can easily
detect a 'bogus' fugitive by his manners," contends
Douglass. The orator concludes that ". . . it is considered bad luck to . . . 'sass' the old folks."

_____. Life and Times of Frederick Douglass
    Written By Himself: His Early Life As A Slave, His
    Escape From Bondage and His Complete History to Pre-
    sent Time. Boston: DeWolfe & Fiske Co., 1892.

(Douglass, Frederick)

The author recalls the influence that his grandmother
had on him during the period that he was a slave. He
states that his grandmother's job was that of baby-
sitter. Douglass surmises that his grandmother's kindness and love stood in place of his mother, whom he
did not know. His aged grandmother, according to the
writer, was a woman of power and spirit.

Hughes, Louis. Thirty Years A Slave: From Bondage to Free-
    dom. The Institution of Slavery as Seen on The Plan-
    tation and in the Home of the Planter. Autobiography
    of Louis Hughes. Milwaukee: South Side Printing Co.,
    1897.

The author states that when a slave woman was too old
to do much of anything, she was assigned to be in
charge of young babies in the absence of their mothers.
He concludes that it was rare that she had any one to
help her.

Langston, John Mercer. From The Virginia Plantation to the
    National Capitol: An Autobiography. Hartford, Conn.:
    American Publishing Co., 1894.

The author pointed out that his master freed in his
will, his aged slaves, including Billy Quarles, who
he also gave two hundred and twenty dollars. Billy
was the oldest and most experienced of the slaves and
was a deeply religious man. The writer also recalls
that Billy was a staunch believer in ghosts. And not
unfrequently, declared Langston, sounds and movements,
which excited his attention and attracted his interest, were ascribed to such agency, at work for man's
good, as he would claim, by appointment of divine Providence. He concludes that had Uncle Billy, as he
called him, not been superstitious, afraid of ghosts,
and easily disturbed by strange noises and curious
sights, so commonly found figuring in the imagination
of the too credulous Virginia slave of the older time,
he would have been by reason of his natural endowments
and general qualities of character, with his experience and observation, eminently successful in any efforts which he might have been called to make in such
capacity.

Northup, Solomon. Twelve Years A Slave: Narrative of
    Solomon Northup, A Citizen of New York, Kidnapped in
    Washington City in 1841, and Rescued in 1853, From a
    Cotton Plantation Near The Red River, in Louisiana.
    Auburn, New York: Derby and Miller, 1853.

The writer points out that aged slaves were patriarchs among other slaves. He recalled "Old Abran was
a kind-hearted being, a sort of patriarch among us,

(Northup, Solomon)

fond of entertaining his younger brethren with grave
and serious discourse. He was deeply versed in such
philosophy as is taught in the cabin of the slave."

Smith, Mrs. Amanda. <u>The Story of The Lord's Dealings With
Mrs. Amanda Smith: An Autobiography</u>. Chicago:
Meyer & Brother, Publishers, 1893.

The writer states that her grandmother was a woman of
deep piety and great faith. She heard her mother
often say that it was to the prayers and mighty faith
of her grandmother that they owed their freedom. The
writer also praised the Lord for a Godly grandmother.
She states that her grandmother often prayed that God
would open a way so that her grandchildren might be
free. Mrs. Smith concludes that tne families into
which these young ladies were to marry, were not considered by the Black folks as good masters and mistresses as they had; and that was one of the grandmother's anxieties. And so she prayed and believed
that somehow God would open a way for their deliver-
ance.

Steward, Austin. <u>Twenty-Two Years A Slave, and Forty Years
A Freeman</u>. Rochester, N. Y.: William Alling, Publisher, 1857.

The author states that on his master's plantation in
Virginia, it was the usual practice to have one of the
old slaves set apart to do the cooking. All field
slaves were required to give into the hands of the
cook a certain portion of their weekly allowance either in dough or meal, which the cook prepared. He
pointed out that his mistress had older servants punished by having them severely whipped by a man, which
she never failed to do for every trifling fault.

2. SLAVE NARRATIVES
COLLECTIONS

Armstrong, Orland Kay. <u>Old Massa's People: The Old Slaves
Tell Their Story</u>. Indianapolis: Bobbs-Merrill Co.,
1931.

The ex-slaves recall that some former aged female
slaves were cooks, seamstresses, weavers and nurses.
They relate that younger slaves learned these and
other "trades" from older slaves.

Egypt, Ophelia Settle, J. Masuoka and Charles S. Johnson,
Editors. <u>Unwritten History of Slavery: Autobiographi-
cal Accounts of Negro Ex-Slaves</u>. Nashville, Tenn.:
Fisk University, Social Science Institute, 1945.

(Egypt, Ophelia S., et al.)

These interviews with ex-slaves were conducted during
1929 and 1930. The subjects resided, for the most
part, in Tennessee and Kentucky. Some ex-slaves recall that they worked some aged slaves almost to death.
Others relate that the aged slave would serve as "doctor" and use homemade remedies and administer them to
the other slaves. Some aged ex-slaves declare that
they went through a lot for young Blacks and that this
later generation should be more appreciative than they
are. Many ex-slaves recollect that their former masters were good to them. Others relate that they were
treated very badly by their former masters. One ex-
slave claimed to be about 120 years old.

Killion, Ronald and Charles Waller, Editors. Slavery
    Time: When I Was Chillun Down on Marster's Planta-
    tion. Savannah, Ga.: Beehive Press, 1973.

This work discusses interviews in Georgia with former
slaves. These interviews were made in the 1930s.
Most of the former slaves were in their eighties' and
nineties'. Some were over one hundred years old.
Many ex-slaves were treated well by their masters,
according to the interviewees.

Perdue, Charles L., Jr., Thomas E. Barden, and Robert K.
    Phillips, Editors. Weevils in the Wheat: Interviews
    with Virginia Ex-Slaves. Charlottesville, Va.: Uni-
    versity Press of Virginia, 1976.

These interviews were conducted during the 1930s as
part of the Virginia Writers' Project. Many of these
former slaves were in their eighties' and nineties'.
A few were over one hundred. Many state that they
were treated kindly by their former masters. Others
declare they were treated very cruelly by their former owners.

Rawick, George P. The American Slave: A Composite Auto-
    biography. Westport, Conn.: Greenwood Press, 1977.
    19 Volumes.

The title tells what this collection is about. These
autobiographies were based on the 1930s Federal Writer's Project interviews. In the 1930s most of these
ex-slaves were in their 80s and 90s. A number were
over 100 years old. They state how they were treated
during slavery. Many recollect that they were treated
kindly by their masters. Others recall that their
masters treated them very cruelly. The ex-slaves
also comment on how aged slaves were treated. Some
were cared for in their old age and others were not.

Tyler, Ronnie C. and Lawrence R. Murphy, Editors. The
    Slave Narratives of Texas. Austin, Tex.: Encino
    Press, 1974.

    The writers' interviews were based mainly on the Feder-
    al Writers' Project collection of the 1930s. Other
    interviews include works found in family papers, and
    archives in libraries in Texas. Most of the ex-slaves
    were in their 80s and 90s in the 1930s. Nearly 25 of
    the 120 interviewed were over 100 years old. Many of
    the ex-slaves stated that they and their families were
    treated well by their former masters. As to be ex-
    pected, most of the aged ex-slaves believed in Jesus
    Christ and were deeply religious. Several had inter-
    esting stories to tell about their childhood experi-
    ences under slavery.

Yetman, Norman R. Life Under The "Peculiar Institution":
    Selection From The Slave Narrative Collection. Hunt-
    ington, N. Y.: Robert E. Krieger Publishing Co.,
    1976.

    These narratives were done in the 1930s by ex-slaves.
    Most of the interviewers were White. These ex-slaves
    were mainly in their 80s and 90s. Several were over
    one hundred years old. One states that he was 125
    years old. Some state they were treated well by their
    masters. Others declare they were treated very cru-
    elly.

3. SLAVE LETTERS

Blassingame, John W., Editor. Slave Testimony: Two Cen-
    turies of Letters, Speeches, Interviews, and Auto-
    biographies. Baton Rouge, La.: Louisiana State Uni-
    versity Press, 1977.

    Various references are made to aged slaves throughout
    this book by former slaves. Many point out that when
    aged slaves could not be of any service to planters,
    they were turned loose upon the mercy of the world.
    Others surmise that the old slaves were generally left
    to sit around in rags and dirt and to take care of the
    children; and when they can not do this, they just lay
    around and suffer, until they die, and there was no
    great account taken of them anyway. Others contend
    that some old slaves were mistreated and abused by
    their masters. There are a few letters from old
    slaves written to their former masters for financial
    assistance. Several newspaper and magazine interviews
    are also included in this collection. Some of the
    slaves and ex-slaves interviewed were eighty and nine-
    ty years old; several were over one hundred years
    old.

Miller, Randall M., Editor. "Dear Master": Letters of A
    Slave Family. Ithaca, N. Y.: Cornell University Press,
    1978.

Various references are made to aged slaves throughout
the book. Some aged slaves were cooks, coachmen, shoe-
makers, preachers, carters, stonemasons, and gardeners.
Some aged slaves mentioned were: "Old" Ben, Judy,
Kessiah Morse, Washington, "Uncle Charles," Etta, etc.

Starobin, Robert S. Black in Bondage: Letters of American
    Slaves. New York: New Viewpoints, 1974.

The letters were written by house servants, drivers,
and artisans who made up an elite group of perhaps 5
or 10 percent of the total slave population. A few
letters were written by ordinary slaves. Many of these
letters were written by aged slaves and refer to aged
slaves. The letters were written in the 1800s. Many
of these letters were written to their masters and former masters by young and aged slaves. Most of the letters were of a complimentary nature. One letter written by an aged female slave stated that she would be
freed by her master if any one would support her.

4.   WHITES' VIEWS OF THE AGED SLAVE

Adams, Nehemiah. South-Side View of Slavery; or Three
    Months At The South. Boston: T. R. Marvin, 1854.

The writer argues that every slave had an inalienable
claim in law upon his owner for support for his whole
life. He states that he observed that on one plantation was a white-headed Black who had done no work for
ten years. The aged slave enjoyed all the privileges
of the plantation, garden, and orchard; he was clothed
and fed as carefully as though he were useful, contends Adams. The author also gives examples of other
aged slaves. Adams points out that one aged slave had
been confined to his bed with rheumatism for thirty
years and was cared for by his master.

Armistead, Wilson, Editor. Five Hundred Thousand Strokes
    For Freedom: A Series of Anti-Slavery Tracts, Of
    Which Half A Million Are Now First Issued By Friends
    of The Negro. London: W. & E. Cash, Publishers, 1853.

Anti-slavery series number 17 is entitled "Sale of
Aged Negroes." This sale took place in Winnsboro,
South Carolina at an auction. An aged male about 70
years old and his wife about the same age were sold
for a meager $13.00. They were almost worn out with
stripes and hard work and both their hair was nearly
white because of old age.

Child, Maria, Editor. <u>The Child's Anti-Slavery Book: Con-
taining A Few Words About American Slave Children and
Stories of Slave-Life</u>. New York: Carlton & Porter,
Publisher, 1859.

One chapter, "Aunt Judy's Story: A Story From Real
Life," by Matilda G. Thompson discusses an aged slave.
The ex-slave told how she was a slave, freed, put back
into slavery and freed again in her old age. She relates how she was "tricked" into slavery by several
planters. Aunt Judy had several children and attempted to find them in her old age, but could not. Unlike some aged slaves, she had no one to depend on in
her old age.

Ingraham, Joseph Hold. <u>The South-West, By a Yankee</u>. New
York: Harper & Brothers, 1835, Vol. 2.

There is one section entitled "Indulgence To Aged
Negroes." The author, a Northerner, traveled in the
Southwest and made the following observations. He
states that aged slaves were sometimes allowed to go
with their children when they were sold, providing
their children would care for them. The author declares "negroes have a peculiarly strong affection
for the old people of their own colour. Veneration
for the aged is one of their strongest characteristics." Ingraham also points out that planters address the aged slaves in a "mild" and "pleasant manner" as "Uncle" or "Aunty"--titles as peculiar to the
old Blacks as "boy" and "girl", to all under forty
years of age. Some aged slaves were allowed to spend
their last years on the master's plantation, without
doing any kind of work. Some, however, did raise a
few vegetables in order to purchase a few extra com-
forts. The author concludes that some planters were
kind to their slaves and indulgenced them.

Lowery, Rev. I. E. <u>Life on The Old Plantation in Ante-
Bellum Days or a Story Based on Facts</u>. Columbia,
S. C.: The State Company, Printers, 1911.

Chapter III is entitled "Granny, The Cook, On The Old
Plantation." The author argues that one of the most
important slaves on this plantation in South Carolina
was Granny, the cook. He points out that she fed,
clothed and raised her master's son and the master's
son "slept in Granny's own bed with his lily white arms
around her black neck." Rev. Lowery concluded that
Granny, though she was Black, considered herself, the
mistress on the plantation because her owner made her
head of the household. The author, eighty years old,
was born on this plantation in 1850, and concludes
that "when Granny gave orders those orders had to be
obeyed. White and Colored respected and obeyed her."

Meade, Bishop. <u>Sketches of Old Virginia Family Servants</u>.
    Philadelphia: Isaac Ashmead, Printer, 1847.

    Various references are made to aged slaves. The
    writer points out that they were nurses and deeply
    religious people. Some could read and write. He sur-
    mises that although some of the aged slaves were in
    their 80s and 90s they still waited on their mistres-
    ses and masters.

Page, Thomas Nelson. <u>The Negro, The Southerner's Problem.</u>
    New York: Charles Scribner's Sons, 1904.

    The author states that as a young lieutenant in a vol-
    unteer company he kissed his old "Black Mammy" on the
    parade ground in sight of the whole company. He
    points out that in one instance, at a wedding in the
    executive mansion at Richmond, Virginia the aged
    slave was left outside and when it was discovered that
    the bride's aged "Mammy" had not come in, the Gover-
    nor himself went out and brought her in on his arm to
    take the place beside the mother of the bride.

_____. <u>Social Life in Old Virginia Before The War</u>.
    New York: Charles Scribner's Sons, 1897.

    The aged slave was the White children's nurse in the
    sense that they were placed in her charge with general
    supervision from the mistress. She also assisted the
    mistress in everything pertaining to the training of
    the children.

Redpath, James. <u>The Roving Editor: Or, Talks with Slaves
    in The Southern States</u>. New York: A. B. Burdick,
    Publisher, 1859.

    The author discusses his talk with an old slave mother
    who was sixty-two. He was shocked because according to
    him, she did not look that old. Redpath points out
    that her maternal affections for her children were
    very strong. The aged slave emphasizes that she and
    other slaves were not contented to be in slavery as
    was reported by White slave owners.

Strother, David Hunter. <u>Virginia Illustrated: Containing
    A Visit to the Virginia Cannan and The Adventures of
    Porte Crayon</u>. New York: Harper and Brothers, 1857.

    The author recalls that when the slave became too old
    for active service, visitors to the plantation came to
    see the old nurse who had been so active in the life
    of the family group. The author argues that it would
    have been an insult both to the aged slave and to the
    family if they did not pay their respects to her. She
    was a personage not to be overlooked, however old she
    might become.

Syrgley, F. D. <u>Seventy Years in Dixie</u>. Nashville, Tenn.:
    Gospel Advocate Publishing Co., 1891.

   The author recalls that for him the aged slave was a
   necessity as his own mother died not long after his
   birth. The aged slave cared for him as a mother would
   and did not give up her tender care until he was
   eighteen years old at which time she died. The author
   states that he was proud of the fact that this slave
   taught him how to count up to ten in an African dia-
   lect.

5. SLAVERY IN THE STATES

Sellers, James Benson. <u>Slavery in Alabama</u>. University,
    Ala.: University of Alabama Press, 1950.

   This work discusses various aspects of aged slaves in
   Alabama. The author repeatedly argues that when
   slaves became old most of them could count on being
   pensioned and allowed to live out their lives without
   working as part of the plantation family. He concludes that "social pressure was brought to bear on
   planters who failed to discharge this part of a slave-
   owner's responsibility." The writer cites several ex-
   cerpts from planters' will books whereby they stated
   that old slaves should be provided for after their
   death.

Smith, Julia Floyd. <u>Slavery and Plantation Growth in Ante-
    bellum Florida, 1821-1860</u>. Gainesville, Fla.: Uni-
    versity of Florida Press, 1973.

   The author points out that the slaves who were too
   old to work in the field were assigned regular duties
   which took less physical effort. Old men worked as
   gardners, wagoners, carters, and stock-tenders. Aged
   women were employed as hospital nurses, assistant
   cooks, workers in the dairy or poultry yard, care-
   takers of Black children in the plantation nursery, or
   in sewing and repairing garments and in spinning and
   weaving. Aged slave women were used as midwives.

Sydnor, Charles Sackett. <u>Slavery In Mississippi</u>. New York:
    D. Appleton-Century Co., 1933.

   The author declares that as slaves grew old, their
   tasks were lightened in proportion to their failing
   strength. He continues to state that on most of the
   larger plantations there were (old) Negroes who either
   did no work or not enough to compensate for their
   food, clothing and shelter. Dr. Sydnor surmises that
   he found no instance of a master's failing to care for
   such slaves and they generally seem to have been treated as well as able-bodied field hands. The writer
   also points out that some planters' wills provided for

(Sydnor, Charles Sackett)

the care or freedom of their aged slaves "who had been faithful for a number of years," or "who have been good, dutiful, and obedient."

Virginia Writers' Project. The Negro in Virginia. New York: Hastings House Publishers, 1940.

Various references are made to aged slaves. Some of the stories are told by former slaves who were now (in 1940) in their 80s and 90s. Others were children and grandchildren of slaves. Some recall the role of the aged slave on the plantation. It was pointed out that it was only on the largest plantations that slave nurses were relieved from other tasks. According to the compilers, to many aged nurses, babies grown to men's estate were still "her children," and even when they became masters of plantations they frequently accorded her the respect and affection due a mother.

6. FEMALE AGED SLAVE

Coffin, Levi. Reminiscences of Levi Coffin, The Reported President of The Underground Railroad. Cincinnati. Robert Clarke Co., 1898.

The author, a White abolitionist, discusses several aged slaves. He mentions one Aunt Betsey, who escapes with her family to freedom. She was a trusty old slave of her master and he reposed considerable confidence in her. She had a husband and eight children. They lived in Kentucky. When Betsey found out that her master intended to sell her children she decided to escape to Ohio, a free state, and this she did. She loaded her family in a wagon, covered them up and pretended to be going to the market in Cincinnati to sell some vegetables. She and her family left and never returned. They later moved to Canada to escape the slave catchers that her former master sent to bring them back.

Doyle, Bertram Wilbur. The Etiquette of Race Relations In The South: A Study in Social Control. Chicago: University of Chicago Press, 1937.

The writer points out that, during slavery the aged female slave's position and relation to the mistress and children were perhaps closer than that of any of the other slaves. According to Doyle she was a kind of "glorified" nurse and was the authority in nursery matters. The younger slave who attended the children as guardian and companion, and who was called "nurse" was subordinate to her. Moreover, it is said, the mistress "humoured her claims of authority," hence the intimacy doubtless begot its own etiquette,

(Doyle, Bertram Wilbur)

concludes the author. Doyle also makes references to
various aged slaves.

Frazier, E. Franklin. The Negro Family in The United
    States. Chicago: University of Chicago Press, 1939.

Chapter 8 is entitled "Granny: The Guardian of The
Generations." Frazier points out that during slavery
the Black grandmother occupied in many instances an
important place in the plantation economy and was
highly esteemed by both the slaves and the masters.
She was the repository of the accumulated lore and
superstition of the slaves and was on hand at the
birth of Black children as well as of White children.
The granny took under her care the orphaned and aban-
doned children. The writer argues that when emancipation came, it was often the old grandmother who kept
the generations together. The Black grandmother's
importance is due to the fact not only that she has
been the "oldest head" in a maternal family organization, but also to her position as "granny" or midwife
among a simple peasant folk, according to the author.
Dr. Frazier concludes that the Black grandmother has
not ceased to watch over the destiny of the Black
families as they moved in ever increasing numbers to
the cities during the 1930s.

Furmas, J. C. Goodbye To Uncle Tom. New York: William
    Sloane Associates, 1956.

Various references are made to the aged slave throughout the book. The author points out that some old
slave women might choose to act as plantation physician, midwife and--more or less secretly--witch doctor.

Goldin, Claudia Dale. Urban Slavery in the American South
    1820-1860: A Quantitative History. Chicago: Univer-
    sity of Chicago Press, 1976.

The writer argues that the 1830 and 1840 urban percentage for older slaves are not much different from
the total United States figures. Some cities, for
example, Norfolk and Richmond, had a slightly older
female slave labor force than the other cities, but
this older age bracket does not, according to Dr.
Goldin, show an abnormal bulge before 1840. The
author concludes that this had changed somewhat by
1850 and differences had become striking by 1860. At
that time all cities except New Orleans had become
older in population by 1860. At that time, argues
Goldin, all cities except New Orleans had a greater
percentage of females older than 54, than did the
United States in general. In some cities, for example,
Norfolk and Washington, the percentage was double that

(Goldin, Claudia Dale)

of the United States.

Murry, Lindley. Narratives of Colored Americans. New York:
    William Wood & Co., 1875.

    Various references are made to aged Blacks throughout
    the book. Most were former slaves. Two particular
    slaves, "Old Dinah" and "Old Susan," stand out. Dinah
    was a slave who was baptized by a Roman Catholic
    priest. She learned to read and was deeply religious.
    Susan also was deeply religious and believed in the
    power of God. Susan was over seventy and she cared
    for her aged mother who was 101 years old.

Myers, Minnie W. Romance and Realism of the South Gulf
    Coast. Cincinnati: Robert Clarke Co., 1898.

    The author points out that the aged slave was the
    first person to whom children visiting the plantation
    ran to see, for she was amiable in her greeting, and
    it was she who saw to all their wants. She showered
    the children with attention and could be kind and in-
    dulgent or stern and exacting as the occasion de-
    manded. The writer declares "Such a thing as rebel-
    lion against her was almost undreamt of, for she was
    high in authority."

Pickens, William. The Heir of Slaves: An Autobiography.
    New York: Pilgrim Press, 1911.

    The author points out that his grandmother lived with
    his mother and father and raised all of the grand-
    children. He recalled that she could thread her own
    needles when she was eighty years old. She lived for
    forty years with a broken back, the upper part of her
    body being carried in a horizontal position, at right
    angles to her lower limbs, so that she had to support
    her steps with a walking cane, if she walked far.
    This was one of the results of slavery. She had been
    beaten and struck across the back with a stick. He
    concludes that even in her old age her temper rose
    quickly, but was volatile and she was a very dear and
    helpful grandmother.

Scarborough, Dorothy. On Trail of Negro Folk-Songs. Cam-
    bridge, Mass.: Harvard University Press, 1925.

    The author tells of an overseer who complained to his
    uncle that the insolence of one of the old women slaves
    was becoming so unbearable that he needed advice about
    punishing her. When told that the old woman's name
    was "Mammy" the uncle replied, "What! What! Why, I
    would as soon think of punishing my own mother! Why
    man you'd have four of the biggest men in Mississippi

(Scarborough, Dorothy)

down on you if you even dare suggest such a thing, and she knows it! All you can do is to knuckle down to Mammy."

Still, William. The Underground Railroad. Philadelphia: Porter & Coates, 1872.

The author alludes to various aged slaves throughout this book. One specific case involves Jane Davis, a slave woman about seventy, from the Eastern Shore section of Maryland. She was the mother of twelve children and "married." Because she was to be sold and often mistreated she decided to leave her children and husband and escape to Buffalo, New York where her brother was living. She escaped by the Underground Railroad. Although she was nearly seventy, she suffered hunger, and slept in the woods for nearly three weeks with little or no food. The author concludes that Jane, doubtless, represented thousands of aged slave mothers, who after having been worn out under the yoke, were frequently either offered for sale for a trifle, turned off to die, or compelled to eke out their existence on the most stinted allowance.

7. TREATMENT OF THE AGED SLAVE

Feldstein, Stanley. Once A Slave: The Slaves' View of Slavery. New York: William Morrow and Co., 1970.

There is one section in this work entitled "The Aged Slave." The author surmises that "one of the shabbier characteristics of slavery described in the slave narratives, and one which tended to deepen the slave's conviction of the infernal character of the institution and to fill him with utter loathing of slaveholders, was the master's alleged lack of gratitude to the aged slave." Prof. Feldstein declares that if no work of any value could be found for them, or if they outlived their original masters and fell into the hands of strangers, they would either be sold for any price they could bring, or simply turned out to fend for themselves. It was pointed out that in some cases of aged slaves being sold for one dollar "to men not worth one cent." In some instances after they had to fend for themselves, some were found starved to death, out of doors, and half eaten up by animals. Some aged slaves became so embittered at being replaced by younger men that their contempt was directed toward their fellow slaves. The author concludes that the elderly slaves were, in the most real sense, the end result of the dehumanization process.

Genovese, Eugene D. Roll, Jordan, Roll: The World The Slaves Made. New York: Pantheon Books, 1974.

(Genovese, Eugene D.)

There is one section entitled "The Old Folks." The
author argues that the reliance of the quarters on
folk medicine gave the old folks a special role--one
that made them feel especially useful and respected
and that brought them a consideration born of religious sanction as well as physical service. The aged
slaves attended the sick, comforted those in pain, and
taught the younger slaves the mysteries of medical
magic. Dr. Genovese contends that suicide appeared
rarely among old slaves. He concludes that the aged
slave had a high degree of security, emotional as well
as physical. Their masters' error, continues the
writer, lay in the supposition that the modest protection of the Big House accounted for their widespread
cheerfulness and contentment, for the old folks' ability to live decently and with self-respect depended primarily on the support of their younger fellow slaves.

Liston, Robert. Slavery in America: The History of
    Slavery. New York: McGraw-Hill Book Co., 1970.

Various references are made throughout the book to
aged slaves. The writer points out that old slaves
had their gray hair dyed black and their silver whis-
kers plucked out to make them appear younger. Liston
contends that planters were ridiculing old slaves when
they called them "auntie" and "uncle." Another form
of ridicule, declares Liston, is when old slave do-
mestics were consulted for their advice on family and
plantation affairs. It was also mentioned by the
author that some old slaves were babysitters and had
other "light" duties to perform.

Owen, Leslie Howard. The Species of Property: Slave Life
    and Culture in The Old South. New York: Oxford Uni-
    versity Press, 1976.

The author asserts that many of the masters assigned
some of the aged light duties such as taking care of
children. Many slaveholders also saw the presence of
some of the old ones as a tax on plantation resources.
Masters emancipated some as a reward for a lifetime of
faithful service, but other planters intended many of
these seeming generosities simply as part of a larger
scheme to set themselves and their relatives free of
responsibility for care of the old persons. The aged
slaves sometimes drifted aimlessly, winding up in
cities where urbanites thought them burdensome additions to the population. Cunning slaveholders doctored
the appearance of the old to make them appear a few
years younger, rested them, and then sold them to anyone who paid a respectable price. The author concludes in all, the aged slave could not look forward to
leisurely final years with certainty. On the larger

(Owen, Leslie Howard)

estates, a planter might be unfamiliar with the care
and food rations actually given to the old ones by
an overseer. If they moved about, he assumed it was
because of age and little else.

Parks, Willis B. The Possibilities Of The Negro in Sym-
posium. Atlanta, Ga.: Franklin Publishing Co., 1904.

There is one article, "Aged Ex-Slaves Gather At Home
Of Old Master," by Robert Timmons included in this
work. Fifteen ex-slaves joined in this reunion in
1899. The oldest member of the party, "Uncle" Edmund
Menefee, who was 80 years old, came from near Hiram,
Georgia, and walked the entire distance, about fifty
miles. They came to see the old homestead and the
other slaves with whom they associated with during
slavery. The author states that the ex-slaves told
of how well they had been treated as slaves and how,
though they wanted freedom, yet when freedom came
they wanted to remain on the same plantation and continue to work for their mistress, after the death of
their master. The ex-slaves also told how their master had taught them to be religious, to be neat and
clean, to be always honest and give the proper respect to the Whites. These lessons, they said, had
remained with them and they were teaching them to
their children.

Stampp, Kenneth M. The Peculiar Institution: Slavery
in The Ante-Bellum South. New York: Alfred A.
Knopf, 1972.

The author argues that a substantial number of aged
"aunties" and "uncles" did not spend their declining
years as pensioners living leisurely and comfortably
on their masters' bounty. A few did, but not enough
reached retirement age to be more than a negligible
expense to the average owner. Dr. Stampp surmises
that doubtless most Blacks in their sixties were not
very productive, but they usually did enough work at
least to pay for their support. Even slaves over
seventy were not always an absolute burden, though it
may be assumed that most were. He concludes that in
1860 only 1.2 percent were over seventy; thus the
owner of as many as a hundred seldom had more than one
or two senile slaves to support.

8. THE BLACK AGED AND THE SLAVERY FAMILY

Gutman, Herbert G. The Black Family In Slavery and Freedom, 1750-1925. New York: Pantheon Books, 1976.

The writer argues that slaves' social beliefs caused
slaves to transfer quickly the names of grandparents

(Gutman, Herbert G.)

to grandchildren. The evidence means that children
often knew their grandparents. This also suggests
that elderly slaves played prominent roles in families formed by their children and especially in socializing and enculturating the young. Gutman concludes that naming practices among plantation slaves
reveal concern for symbolic ties to older Black kin.

Webber, Thomas L. Deep Like the Rivers: Education in the
    Slave Quarter Community, 1831-1865. New York: W.
    W. Norton & Co., 1978.

Chapter 13 is entitled "The Family." The author declares that although aged slaves maintained their own
cabins until death, the general rule in most quarter
communities was for single aged slaves to move in with
one of their married children after they became too
old to work in the fields. Respected for their age
and for their position as head of the family, grandparents often enjoyed a venerated authority in the
family. In most quarter families, states Webber,
children learned that when their family gathered together, it was the commands of grandparents that were
to be obeyed first. Often one or more grandparents
assumed the role of the arbiter in family disputes
and quarrels. The author concludes that grandparents
also played an important educational role in transmitting the songs and stories of Africa and of plantation history. One of childhood's chief diversions,
according to the writer, was to listen to the songs
and tales of grandparents.

    9. ECONOMIC VALUE OF THE BLACK AGED

Catterall, Helen Tunncliff, Editor. Judicial Cases Con-
    cerning American Slavery and The Negro. Washington,
    D. C.: Carnegie Institution of Washington, 1936.
    Vol. 2, pp. 101-102, 186-187.

The editor lists two cases relating to aged Blacks in
North Carolina. They are: Lane v. Wingate, 3 Iredell
326, June 1843 [327] "the plaintiff declined selling
him, alleging that he wanted Daniel to wait upon an
old negro woman. . . named Rhoda, who was upwards of
one hundred years of age, . . . defendant replied,
that if the plaintiff would let him have Daniel, he
would support old Rhoda during her life; the parties
valued Daniel at two hundred dollars, and the defendant executed the agreement." Rhoda remained with
the defendant [327] for about four weeks, after which
time she returned to the house of the plaintiff, where
she has remained ever since. . . it was worth twenty-
five dollars a year to support Rhoda. . . [328] ver-
dict for the plaintiff, assessing his damages at

(Catterall, Helen Tunncliff)

seventy-five dollars." The other case includes
Joiner v. Joiner, 2 Jones Eq. 68, December 1854.
Will: [69] "to my son Noah. . . the cooper Joseph,
. . . and James." Codicil, three years later: "that
Robert Hines have . . . the boy James." The testator
owned two negroes by the name of James: "one. . .
was a valuable young man. The other . . . was very
old, supposed to be near one hundred, and not only
without value, but an expense." Held: "we cannot
. . . believe that a father would mock his son by
giving him, as an apparent bounty, an old negro, who
was . . . a burden."

Davis, Edwin Adams, Editor. Plantation Life in Florida
Parishes of Louisiana, 1836-1846 As Reflected in The
Diary of Bennet H. Barrow. New York: Columbia Uni-
versity Press, 1943.

Under the "Rules of Highland Plantation," the planter
stated that if a slave would work for him until he
got old and could no longer maintain himself, then
he would care for him. In the 1855 "Inventory of the
Estate of Bennet H. Barrow," it listed several aged
slaves and their value: Betsy age 59, $100.00; Old
Sukey age 56, $100.00; Lucy, age 71, only $10.00;
Dennis, age 44, $150.00; Josh, age 69, $100.00; Phil,
age 75, $100.00; Old Hannah, age 70, only $5.00; Old
Cato, age 60, $400.00; Judis, age 56, $100.00; Ceely,
age 54, $100.00. This book also gives "Slave Deaths:
1831-1845." Two slaves, Old Pat, age 80 and Old Jack
age 85 died 1831, and 1834 respectively. Two other
slaves, Old Rheuben, age 60 and Old Betty, age 65,
both died in 1836.

Fogel, Robert William and Stanley L. Engerman. Time On
The Cross: The Economics of American Negro Slavery.
Boston: Little, Brown and Co., 1974.

Various references are made to the economic status of
aged slaves. The authors argue that earnings of
sixty-five year olds were still positive and on an
average, brought owners as much net income as a
slave in the mid-teens. They declare that the above
statement does not mean that every slave aged sixty-
five produced a positive net income for his owner.
Some of the elderly, according to Fogel and Engerman,
were a net loss. However, the income earned by the
able-bodied among the elderly was more than enough to
compensate for the burden imposed by the incapaci-
ted, conclude the authors. The writers state that
fully 40 percent of the slaves died before age nineteen.

10.   THE BLACK AGED SLAVE AS A STORYTELLER

Dundes, Alan, Editor.   Mother Wit From the Laughing Barrel.
Englewood Cliffs, N. J.:   Prentice Hall, Inc., 1973.

Various references are made to the Black aged throughout this book on Black Folklore.   One section of particular interest is "Dialogues of The Old and The
New Porter."   This is a conversation between a young
Black pullman porter and an elderly Black porter.   The
young Black convinced the aged Black porter to join
the Pullman Sleeping Car Porters' Union.   Another
section, "Old-Time Courtship Conversation," discusses
the Black aged.   This essay discusses "courtship" of
slaves on plantations.   The author states that almost
every large plantation had an experienced old slave
who instructed young slaves in the way in which they
should go in the delicate matter of winning the girls
of their choice.   This is what this work is about.

Levine, Lawrence W.   Black Culture and Black Conscience:
Afro-American Folk Thought From Slavery To Freedom.
New York: Oxford University Press, 1977.

The writer makes various references to the Black
aged.   He points out that on some plantations, the
aged Black slaves were "doctors" or "root doctors"
who used herbs and "roots" as medicine.   A number of
slave practitioners won considerable renown for their
skill.   In 1729 the governor of Virginia traded an
elderly slave "who has performed many wonderful cures
of diseases" his freedom in return for the secret
of his medicine, "a concoction of roots and barks."
The writer also relates that old slaves had signs for
everything.   These were signs indicating what the
weather would be; signs telling of the coming of
strangers or loved ones; signs prophesying bad luck
or good fortune; signs warning of an impending whip-
ping or the approach of white patrols; signs fore-
telling imminent illness or death.   Dreams were taken
seriously as an important source of such signs, concludes the writer.

11.   BLACK AGED AND RELIGION

Henderson, Donald H.   The Negro-Freedman: Life Conditions
of the American Negro in the Early Years After Emancipation.   New York: Henry Schuman, 1952.

The author discusses aged Blacks and their views on
education, superstitions and religion.   It was pointed
out that aged Blacks went to public schools to acquire
an education.   The old people wanted to learn to read
the Bible before they died, and wished their children
to be educated.   Dr. Henderson states that an inves-
tigator reported having seen three generations--a

(Henderson, Donald H.)

grandmother, a daughter, and a granddaughter--sitting on the same bench, spelling the same lesson, and having seen classes that included pupils from six years of age up to sixty. The aged also were deeply superstitious and religious.

Herskovits, Melville J. The Myth of The Negro Past. New York: Harper and Brothers, 1941.

The author points out that one of the things that slaves brought to America from Africa was their respect for their elders. He states that the early slaves in America referred to their elders as "almost ghosts." Herskovits declares that the validity of this explanation is best indicated by referring the assertion that "old folks" are "almost ghosts" to the tenets of the ancestral cult which, as one of the most tenacious Africanisms, has left many traces in the New World Negro customs. He continues to state the belief in the power of the ancestors to help or harm their descendants in a fundamental sanction of African relationship groupings, and this has influenced the retention of Africanisms in many aspects of Negro life in the New World.

Miller, Harriet Parks. Pioneer Colored Christians. Clarksville, Tenn.: W. P. Titus, Printer, 1911.

This book includes the Christian views of ex-slaves. They were born between 1810 and 1850. Most of these aged Blacks state that they never would have reached old age except for the grace and will of God. He was the one that carried them through.

Woofter, Thomas J., Jr. Black Yeomanry: Life on St. Helena Island. New York: Henry Holt and Co., 1930.

The author states that there are many ex-slaves who are near ninety. He argues this longevity is in itself a striking commentary on the health of the Island. He concludes that theirs is not a bedridden old age and seldom are they entirely dependent. Many of the old men and old women, according to the writer, are straight as a string and do occasional field work or odd jobs up to the time of their last illness. The ex-slaves were also deeply religious people.

Articles

1. FEMALE AGED SLAVE

Brown, Clarence. "Reflections on 119 Years of Living,"
     <u>Jet</u>, July 4, 1974, pp. 22-25.

   Article concerns Mrs. Mary Mood, born a slave on an
   Augusta, Arkansas plantation almost 10 years before
   the signing of the Emancipation Proclamation. She
   has been called the "oldest Black woman in the United
   States." Mrs. Mood has lived under the rule of 23
   presidents. She gives her views on sex, President
   Nixon, her longevity, the moon landing, today's fashions, airplanes, and food prices.

Flander, Ralph B. "Two Plantations in a County of Ante-
     bellum Georgia," <u>Georgia Historical Quarterly</u>, Vol.
     7, March, 1928, pp. 1-24.

   The writer points out that aged, infirm or crippled
   slaves wove baskets, mended or made clothes, or were
   assigned light tasks about the place. The old women
   often canned fruit and cared for the children.

Jacobs, Harriet. "The Good Grandmother" in <u>The Freed-
     men's Book</u>, L. Maria Child, Editor. Boston: Tick-
     nor and Fields, 1865, pp. 206-218.

   The writer, a slave, states that her grandmother was
   a remarkable woman in many respects. Her grandmother,
   also a slave, made enough money baking crackers at
   night to purchase the freedom of her children. The
   grandmother was purchased for fifty dollars by an
   old White lady who gave her her freedom. The author,
   who also gained her freedom, along with her grandmother moved to the North.

Parkhurst, Jessie W. "The Role of The Black Mammy in the
     Plantation Household," <u>Journal of Negro History</u>,
     Vol. 23, No. 3, July, 1938, pp. 349-369.

(Parkhurst, Jessie W.)

Various references are made to the aged "Black Mammy."
The author points out that she was considered self-
respecting, independent, loyal, forward, gentle, cap-
tious, affectionate, true, strong, just, warm-hearted,
compassionate-hearted, fearless, popular, brave, good,
pious, quick-witted, capable, thrifty, proud, regal,
courageous, superior, skillful, tender, queenly, dig-
nified, neat, quick, competent, possessed with a tem-
per, trustworthy, faithful, patient, tyrannical, sen-
sible, discreet, efficient, careful, harsh, devoted,
truthful, neither apish nor servile. The aged mammy,
according to the author, was a diplomat and knew how
to handle delicate situations with such a fine sense
of appropriateness that her purpose was usually accom-
plished. From being a confidential servant she grew
into being a kind of prime minister, states the writer.
The writer states that it was well known that if she
espoused a cause and took it to the master it was
sure to be attended to at once, and according to her
advice. The aged Black Mammy was at the top of the
social hierarchy of slaves and occupied a position
to be envied as well as to be strived for. The old
Black Mammy was skillful in making old home remedies
and upon them the White plantation had to depend
when medicine gave out and no more was to be had, concludes the author.

2.   TREATMENT OF THE AGED SLAVE

Corlew, Robert E. "Some Aspects of Slavery in Dickson
    County (Tennessee)," _Tennessee Historical Quarterly_,
    Vol. 10, 1951, pp. 224-248, 344-365.

The author argues that occasionally, if a slave was
old, the owner would provide for both emancipation
and support in old age. Such was the case with John
Humphries and many others. Humphries in 1826 provided in his will that "my old negro woman Amy . . .
is to be permitted to live with which of my children
she pleases but not as a slave, and which ever she
chooses to live with shall be bound to maintain her
as long as she lives . . . ."

"In The South The Slaves Are Taken Care Of for Past Ser-
    vices," _New York Herald Tribune_, March 8, 1860, p. 4.

Article discusses four old Black slave pensioners in
Alabama. One was eighty years old. Another one was
seventy-five years old. The other two were fifty
years old. The writer states that all four were well
taken care of by their masters.

3. HISTORICAL PERSPECTIVES OF THE BLACK AGED

Blassingame, John W.   "Status and Social Structure in The
    Slave Community: Evidence From New Sources." Per-
    spectives and Irony in American Slavery. Harry P.
    Owens, Editor. Jackson, Mississsippi: University
    Press of Mississippi, 1976, pp. 137-151.

    The author makes various references to aged slaves.
    He points out that aged slaves were deeply religious
    and they stressed the importance of it on young
    slaves. Old slaves also taught young male slaves the
    "proper" formula of "courtship." Aged slaves accord-
    ing to the writer, often demonstrated their verbal
    skills at church. One of the primary marks of a
    slave's piety was his or her ability to bear public
    witness to God in the form of prayer. Religious testi-
    mony was so important, states Dr. Blassingame, that
    slaves reduced prayers to formulas and taught them to
    young converts. Aged slaves also carved exquisite
    walking canes or whistles for youngsters and slave
    women were skillful seamstresses and made beautiful
    quilts. The author surmises that old men and women
    with great stores of riddles, proverbs, and folktales
    played a crucial role in teaching morality and train-
    ing the young to solve problems and to develop their
    memories. Age gradations represent one of the keys to
    social structure with elders being viewed as the pos-
    sessors of wisdom, the closest link to the African
    homeland, and persons to be treated with respect, con-
    cludes the author.

Wylie, Floyd M. "Attitude Toward Aging Among Black Ameri-
    cans: Some Historical Perspectives." Aging and Human
    Development, Vol. 2, 1971, pp. 66-70.

    The writer surmises that fortunately many of the cul-
    tural values and attitudes regarding the elderly have
    apparently changed little over the several centuries
    since Africans were snatched from their home continent.
    Wylie contends that the period of the slave trade and
    slavery did not divest Africans and their descendants
    of many basically African cultural values. The author
    concludes that it is clear that among the more impor-
    tant of these values that continue to the present time
    are a certain respect and even veneration of age, and
    frequently strikingly different attitudes about the
    aging process and the role and place of older persons
    within the culture. He also states this historical
    perspective will hopefully provide a different under-
    standing, appreciation, and recognition of the essen-
    tially humanitarian view that Black Americans take of
    their older folk.

2.

MAJOR
BOOKS

Bell, Duran, et al. <u>Delivering Services To Elderly Members of Minority Groups: A Critical Review Of The Literature</u>. Santa Monica, Calif.: The Rand Corp., April, 1976.

One of the authors' avowed objectives was "to improve future research in such a way that it will be more useful to public policy." The authors in their review of the literature conclude that race may be important in the design and implementation of a service delivery system for elderly and nonelderly Blacks; the relevance of race arises however not from the higher incidence of Blacks among lower socioeconomic categories but because of the cultural, historical and educational factors that affect the extent to which race neutral programs can be effective in actually providing services to similarly situated persons from different racial groups. The authors criticize Black researchers when they argue: "The promotion of research on problems of the Black elderly has tended to rest on the claim that Black elderly have qualitatively different problems than other groups. The contention is that Black elderly have unique problems and needs that should be studied separately perhaps in the context of special institutes or training programs. But if it turns out that apparent race differences are simply a function of the differences in the distribution of racial groups across SES categories, the special significance of research on Black elderly would be less compelling." The authors went on to state that the literature fails to define any problems that would indicate a need for methods of service delivery unique to Blacks and that although it may be useful to know that the average Black is poorer than the average non-Black, such information has little or no bearing on a service delivery process except to imply that Blacks need more of such services, conclude the authors.

Chan, Peter, Editor. <u>Reading In Black Aged</u>. New York:
    MSS Information Corp., 1977.

This is a collection of twenty-two previously published articles. Of this number, seven are by Jacquelyne Johnson Jackson, the leading authority on the
Black Aged. These essays deal with four areas: over-
view, research, services and social policy. Most of
the articles have appeared in <u>Aging and Human Devel-</u>
<u>opment</u>, <u>Proceedings of Research Conference on Minor-</u>
<u>ity Groups Aged in The South</u>, <u>Gerontologist</u>, <u>Phylon</u>,
and <u>Family Coordinator</u>.

Dancy, Joseph, Jr. <u>The Black Elderly: A Guide For Prac-</u>
    <u>titioners</u>. Ann Arbor, Mich.: The Institute of Ger-
    ontology, University of Michigan-Wayne State Univer-
    sity, 1977.

This book discusses the following major points: (1)
raise the consciousness of practitioners and their
employing institutions and agencies in regard to the
particular needs, problems, and strengths of the
Black elderly; (2) suggest how the Black elderly can
be served more appropriately and supportively; (3)
provide the practitioner with a better understanding
of the cultural heritage and traditions of the Black
elderly; and (4) encourage the practitioner to reexamine his or her own attitudes about aging and minorities. The author also gives some of the strengths
of the Black elderly: (1) an accumulation of wisdom,
knowledge, and common sense about life that comes
not only from age, but from their particular experience of hardship and suffering; (2) they have a creative genius in doing much with little; (3) their ability to accept their own aging and regarding old age
as a reward in itself; (4) they hold a sense of hope
and optimism for a better day, in spite of a past full
of hardships. Dancy concludes that in these strengths
of good sense and resourcefulness, acceptance and
hope, elderly Blacks offer an inspiration for us all.
This work has a comprehensive bibliography and appen-
dixes that include some institutions with special concerns for the Black elderly and selected films and
videotapes.

Davis, Frank G. <u>The Black Community's Social Security</u>.
    Washington, D. C.: University Press of America, 1978.

This book is designed to test and evaluate the validity and the social security implications of the author's basic hypothesis of declining personal income
of the lower income masses of the Black community
relative to the income of the White community, and to
demonstrate the resultant permanent high incidence of
poverty and personal income insecurity in the Black
community, notwithstanding the insurance provisions

(Davis, Frank G.)

of the present Social Security Act. The author concludes: (1) Old-age insurance tax costs in the Black
community substantially exceed old-age insurance benefits; (2) Old-age insurance benefits payable to the
Black community are far below the poverty level; when
at the same time, almost two-fifths of Blacks age 65
and over are below the poverty level as compared to
only 14 percent of Whites; (3) Over-all rises in
Social Security benefits, accruing to the Black community are more than washed out by ultimate rises in
Social Security taxes.

Jackson, Jacquelyne Johnson, Editor. Proceedings of The
Research Conference on Minority Group Aged in the
South. Durham, N. C.: Center for the Study of Aging
and Human Development, Duke University Medical Center,
1972.

Twenty-two papers are discussed in this collection.
There are also four major Appendices: (1) Selected
Statistical Data on Aging and Aged Blacks; (2) Profile of Aged Blacks in Nonmetropolitan Areas: Statistical Tabulations; (3) Aged Blacks: A Selected
Bibliography; (4) Selected Bibliography on the Aged
in Ethnic Minorities. This conference focused upon
completed, on-going, and needed research on Black
aged. Its major purposes--examining the current status of research on Black aged, with special emphasis
upon identifying critical research gaps, and encouraging more research--to investigate carefully Black
aged--can best be realized through significant increases in such researches and researchers as direct
or indirect outgrowths of this Conference concludes
the editor of these papers.

_____, Editor. Proceedings of Conference on Black
Aged in The Future. Durham: Center For the Study
of Aging and Human Development, Duke University, 1973.

The title tells what this 140 page book is about.
The topics include "Black Aged in the Future in a
Predominantly Black Southern Town," by Johnny Ford;
"Death and Dying: A Cross-Cultural View," by
Richard A. Kalish; "Housing and Geriatric Centers
For Aging and Aged Blacks," by Hobart C. Jackson;
"Housing For the Aged Blacks," by Abraham Isserman;
"Medical Aspects of The Aged American Black," by
Nathaniel O. Calloway; "Dental Health of Aged Blacks"
by Reginald A. Hawkins; "Nursing Care of the Aged,"
by Jeanne J. Penn; "The Future of The Black Aged in
America," by Charles H. Palm; "A Psychiatric Strategy
for Aged Blacks in The Future," by James H. Carter;
"Curriculum Development on Aged Blacks in Predomi-
nantly White Environments," by Walter Beattie and

(Jackson, Jacquelyne Johnson)

Harry Morgan; and "Social Stratification of Aged
Blacks and Implications For Training Professionals,"
by Jacquelyne J. Jackson, the editor of these proceedings.

_____. Minorities and Aging. Belmont, Calif.: Wads-
worth Co., 1980.

This is the latest and most complete work on minorities and aging by the leading authority on Black Aging. Much of this book deals with the Black aged.
The basic theme on Black aged is that they have special and unique needs that must be met by aggressive
programs by the federal, state and local governments.
Some attention is also devoted to the role of the
National Center On The Black Aged.

National Urban League. Double Jeopardy, The Older Negro
in America Today. New York: National Urban League,
1964.

The League states that aged Blacks are in "double jeopardy" because they are (in 1964) the most desperate
of any American group. Moreover, it argues that
"Today's (1964) aged Negro is different from today's
White because he is a Negro." This organization went
on to point out that since 10.5% of White old-age-
assistance recipients in a national study were found
to be institutionalized, then 10.5% of the Negro recipients, rather than 2.4% as was the case, should
also have been institutionalized. Some writers dis-
agree with this theory.

Pollard, Lu Lu. Retirement--Black and White. New York:
Exposition Press, Inc., 1973.

The author discusses the retirement of the Black aged
with the White aged. She compares certain facets of
retirement such as "Fears of Retirement," "Retirement
Income," "Retirement Housing," "The Counselor's Role,"
and "The Role of the Community." The concluding chapter is entitled "White vs. Black Retirement." The
writer asserts that too frequently the Black retiree
must seek aid from welfare, not because he does not
want to work, but because he was for so many years
denied an opportunity to earn a decent livelihood,
which would be reflected in his retirement pension.
She concludes that the Black worker has been denied
knowledge that could help him in retirement because
no one in management thought it important to prepare
him for retirement in the same way that the White
worker was prepared.

Stanford, E. Percil, Editor. Institute Proceedings on
     Minority Aging and The Legislative Process. San
     Diego, Calif.: Center on Aging, San Diego State
     University, 1977.

     The title tells what this book is about. The follow-
     ing topics are discussed: "Strategies For Effective
     Input By The Elderly," "Historical and Current Per-
     spectives on Legislation," "Role of the Regional
     Office," "Policy Issues and The Minority Aged," "Over-
     view of Policy Issues and Their Impact on the Ethnic
     Elderly," "Policy and the Minority Aged," "Policy and
     the Minority Aged at the State Level," "The Minority
     Aging--An Action," "Retirement Legislation and The
     Minority Aged," "Strategies For Affecting Legislative
     Priorities," "Social Security and Supplemental In-
     come," "The State Office on Aging and Legislative Im-
     plications," and "Political Consideration For Change."
     There is also a good Bibliography and Appendices.

_____. The Elder Black: A Cross-Cultural Study of
     Minority Elders in San Diego. San Diego: Center on
     Aging, San Diego State University, 1978.

     This work deals with three specific objectives. First,
     it analyzes characteristic lifestyles and customs, as
     well as the primary interactional networks of ethnic
     minority groups and in this case, especially those of
     Black elders. Second, it explores and delineates the
     perceptions and viewpoints of the Black elders toward
     formal programmatic assistance and human service net-
     works with the overall intent of tracing, where possi-
     ble, the interactions between the formal programs and
     the primary networks. Third, it tested out a method-
     ology appropriate to obtaining information about eth-
     nic minority populations and specifically the elders
     of these populations. The writer concludes that gen-
     erally, the findings in this study indicate that the
     services available and the services actually used by
     the elderly Blacks in the sample are two divergent
     issues. Services are often available and may even be
     accessible. The reality is that too many of the el-
     derly in the sample were not aware of the specifics
     of the services and had they been aware, many would
     have, in fact, used some of the services. This work
     has an annotated bibliography on Black Aging and also
     other works on Black Aging.

Watson, Wilbur, et al., Editors. Health and The Black Aged.
     Washington, D. C.: National Center on Black Aged,
     1978.

     The title tells what this work is about. The follow-
     ing topics were discussed: "The Study of Hyperten-
     sion Compliance in a Group of Elderly Third World
     Patients," "Carcinoma of the Prostate Gland in

(Watson, Wilbur, et al.)

California: A Candid Look at Survival Trends in Re-
gards to Stage, Race, and Social Class," "Health Indicators and Life Expectancy of the Black Aged: Policy Implications," "Mobility Among The Physically Impaired Black Aged," "Doctor Can't Do Me No Good:
Social Concomitants of Health Care Attitudes and Practices Among Elderly Blacks in Isolated Rural Populations," "Poverty, Folk Remedies and Drug Misuse Among
The Black Elderly," "Perceived Health Status of the
Black Elderly in an Urban Area: Findings of a Survey
Research Project," "Ethnicity and Aging in Elderly
Black Women: Some Mental Health Characteristics,"
"The Social Psychology of Black Aging: The Effects
of Self-Esteem and Perceived Control on The Adjust-
ment of Older Black Adults," "Health Status of a Suc-
cessful Black Aged Population Related to Life Satis-
faction and Self-Concept," "The Aged and Aging Black
Prison Inmate: An Inquiry into Some Mental Health
Consequences of Imprisonment," "A Community-Based,
Consumer Controlled, Comprehensive Approach to Health
Care for the Black Elderly," and "Medical Screening
Project: One Answer to a City's Problem."

3.

GENERAL
BOOKS

1. BLACK AGED AND CHILDREN

Harrison-Ross, Phyliss and Barbara Wyden. The Black Child:
    A Parent's Guide. New York: Berkley Medallion Book,
    1973.

    Chapter 33 is entitled "What Grandma Doesn't Know."
    The authors surmise that what the older generation of
    Blacks doesn't know about cuddling--If you don't re-
    spond to a young child's needs, he won't respond to
    you and others later. The writers state, "Don't ex-
    pect the older generation to accept all new ideas."
    The authors argue that in many cases Black mothers de-
    pend on grandmothers to discipline and help raise their
    children.

Hill, Robert B. The Strengths of Black Families. New
    York: Emerson Hall Publisher, 1971.

    In Part 1 of this work there is one section entitled
    "Absorption of Individuals: Minors and the Elderly."
    The writer contends that the families headed by elder-
    ly Black women take in the highest proportion (48 per-
    cent) of children. He declares that about the same
    proportion of Black and White families have elderly
    persons living with them, except in families headed by
    a woman where a higher proportion of White (10 percent)
    than Black (4 percent) families had elderly members.
    These elderly persons play important roles in many of
    these families such as baby-sitting with grandchildren.
    These services often provide additional income to el-
    derly persons. Dr. Hill concludes that elderly Black
    women are more likely to take children into their own
    households than be taken into the household of younger
    kin.

Lewis, Hylan. Blackways of Kent. Chapel Hill, N. C.: Uni-
    versity of North Carolina Press, 1950.

(Lewis, Hylan)

The writer argues that in general, the attitude of Black young people toward the Black aged is one of respect and kindness; there tends to be marked filial respect and obedience among all groups. The author concludes that a significant amount of the respect for the older persons is related to the following facts: they control a significant part of the wealth or means of support as propertied heads of families or widows, and; pension payments give many a measure of support and release them from dependence upon relatives or friends. The older Blacks play another important role in Kent society; they are not only significant links with the ways of previous generations of Kent Blacks, but they are also significant links with present and past generations of Kent Whites.

Martin, Elmer P. and Joanne Michell Martin. The Black Extended Family. Chicago: University of Chicago Press, 1978.

Chapter Five is entitled "Relations Between Old and Young Child Rearing" and discusses the Black elderly. The authors point out that the Black aged extended family member, believing that the "old fashioned" ways of preparing young members for living in America have made for the maintenance of the family and the welfare of its members, seek to impart those ways to the young. The writers see the Black aged, though still among the most respected individuals in the extended family, experiencing a sense of uneasiness as, day after day, they see their roles as child raisers diminish. The educators conclude that the Black aged are finding it more difficult to have an impact on the lives of their extended families as the mass media, peer-group influence, the educational system, and a mechanistic conformity to fads and fashions push their influence further into the background. To the Black aged, those old-fashioned ways of reacting to oppression by patience, by indirection, and by perseverance, are the cornerstone of Black extended family stability. When members of their extended family reject the time-proven ways of confronting life, the aged reproach them for rejecting their truest heritage, conclude the authors.

Powdermaker, Hortense. After Freedom: A Cultural Study in The Deep South. New York: Atheneum, 1969.

The author points out that grandmothers are present in many households, and are likely to loom larger than mothers on the child's horizon, even when the real mother retains the chief authority. She also states that, frequently, they are at home when the mother goes out to work, although, because of the

(Powdermaker, Hortense)

early marriages, the grandmother too is often young enough for strenuous labor. Where an elderly woman is head of a household, including married daughters, she carries authority with the children; and even where her position is less dominant, she is likely to take over a share of responsibility for their welfare and behavior, concludes the writer.

Stack, Carol B. <u>All Our Kin: Strategies For Survival in a Black Community</u>. New York: Harper and Row, Publishers, 1974.

Various references are made to Black grandmothers and Black grandfathers. It is pointed out that many Black children are raised by their grandmothers. Many of these grandparents live with their children and grandchildren.

Staples, Robert. <u>Introduction To Black Sociology</u>. New York: McGraw Hill Book Co., 1976.

There is one section on "The Aged." The author states that in most cases, the grandmothers are more likely to take children into their own households than to be taken into the household of their kinfolk. Dr. Staples argues that about half (48 percent) of elderly Black women have other related children living with them--in contrast to only 10 percent of similar White families. He concludes that this is but one more indication of the strong cohesiveness and prevalent concern for one another within Black families. Most aged Black parents desire to live independently of, but in close contact with, their children.

Wright, Richard. <u>Black Boy: A Record of Childhood and Youth</u>. New York: Harper & Brothers, 1945.

The author discusses the many conflicts that he had with his grandmother during his childhood. She was a deeply religious woman and attempted to convert him to her faith. This he refused to do. Although he was raised partly by his grandmother, Wright had many disagreements with her. He did, however, love her very much. He did what was almost unheard of in the Black community and that was to speak up and disobey his grandmother's wishes.

2. BLACK AGED AND THE BLACK FAMILY

Bernard, Jessie. Marriage and Family Among Negroes.
    Englewood Cliffs, N. J.: Prentice-Hall, Inc., 1966.

> The author asserts that the position of the oldest wo-
> man in a family was, traditionally, an extremely im-
> portant one: it was she, not the male head of the
> family, who had the role of the matriarch. Dr. Ber-
> nard argues that the grandmother played an important
> part even during slavery, "highly esteemed by both
> the slaves and the masters." Often she was the con-
> fidential adviser of the older members of the slave
> household. Moreover, age added "dignity" to her posi-
> tion and "her regime." The writer concludes that
> these "grannies" were genuine matriarchs--powerful
> stabilizing figures who performed a profoundly impor-
> tant service--but they have all but disappeared from
> the scene.

Billingsley, Andrew. Black Families In White America.
    Englewood Cliffs, N. J.: Prentice-Hall, Inc., 1968.

> Various references are made throughout the book about
> the Black aged in Africa, during the slavery era, and
> in present day American society. The author points out
> the influence that various Black aged middle class
> had on the children and grandchildren. Some of the
> aged families discussed include the Hildrus Poindexter
> family, the Langston Hughes family and the Martin Lu-
> ther King family.

Birmingham, Stephen. Certain People: America's Black
    Elite. Little, Brown, and Co., 1977.

> Part Three, "The Old Guard," is a discussion of aged
> Blacks. They prefer "Negro." Most of the aged Black
> elite are proud of their family backgrounds, accord-
> ing to the author.

Haley, Alex. Roots: The Saga of An American Family. New
    York: Doubleday & Co., 1974.

> Aged Blacks and the role they played in Africa, slave
> family and freed family are discussed throughout this
> classic. Some of the aged include Grandmother Yaisa,
> Juffure's Council of Elders, Omoro, Binta Nyo Boto,
> Old Fiddler, Kizzy, Will Palmer, etc. He discusses
> the influence that aged Blacks had on him and other
> Blacks throughout history.

Kennedy, Carroll E. Human Development: The Adult Years
    and Aging. New York: Macmillan Publishing Co., 1978.

> There is one section in this work that deals with the
> Black families. The author points out that the fact

(Kennedy, Carroll E.)

that there are few Blacks in nursing homes suggests
something of the nature of the extended-family concept in the Black community. Moreover, many Black
families take relatives into their households. These
relatives, however, are more likely to be children
than older relatives. Older women tend to take in
children and younger persons rather than being taken
in themselves.

Sager, Clifford J., Thomas L. Brayboy, and Barbara R. Wax-
    enberg. Black Ghetto Family in Therapy: A Labora-
    tory Experience. New York: Grove Press, 1970.

One Black grandmother was discussed in this book. It
was pointed out that the Black grandmother was not
the domineering force in the Black family. The authors surmise that in many cases the Black grandmother does not want to dominate the family, she only
wants to be included in it; to feel as though she's
important.

3.   BLACK AGED FEMALES

Carson, Josephine. Silent Voices: The Southern Negro
    Woman Today. New York: Dell Publishing Co., 1969.

This book is based on interviews of several Black
women throughout the South; some were Black aged.
The women tell what they think and feel--about themselves, their futures, their religions, their friends,
their employers, their leaders, about their politics
or lack of them, about segregation and integration,
about White people and White culture, about love and
old age and death, above all, about human dignity.
The author points out that in 1968 seventy-five percent of aged Black women lived alone. Ninety-six
percent had less than $2,000 a year to live on. Six-
ty-eight percent had less than $1,000 a year. Sever-
al aged Black women that Miss Carson interviewed fall
in the above category.

DuBois, W. E. Burghardt. Dusk of Dawn: An Essay Toward
    An Autobiography of Race Concept. New York: Har-
    court, Brace & World, Inc., 1940.

The author discusses his grandmother and grandfather.
He states they raised him and influenced him greatly.
Dr. DuBois surmises that with Africa he had only one
direct cultural connection and that was the African
melody which his great-grandmother violently used to
sing.

Wembridge: Elanor Rowland. Life Among the Lowbrows.
    Boston: Houghton Mifflin Co., 1931.

(Wembridge, Elanor Rowland)

The writer, who is White, points out that the Black grandmothers take better care of themselves in their old age than the White grandmothers. The Black female elderly women see themselves as independent individuals able to take care of themselves. The author concludes that of all old women, the Black aged represent the eternal feminine. The Black aged, according to the writer, have drunk from the fountain of youth and have never lost its flavor. She also states that the Black aged has dignity.

4.   BLACK AGED POPULATION

Brotman, Herman B.   Facts and Figures on Older Americans. Washington, D. C.: Administration on Aging, No. 2, 1971, p. 3.

The writer points out that shorter life expectancy for Negroes produces a smaller proportion of older persons. The 22.7 million Negroes of all ages represent 11.2% of the total resident population. The older Negro population increased from 1.2 million in 1960 to 1.6 million in 1970 and, since this was a higher rate of growth than that of the total Negro population, they made up 6.9% of all Negroes as compared with 6.2% in 1960. Like the White population, moreover, the older women outnumber the older men and the discrepancy is increasing. The ratio of women per 100 men among 65+ Negroes rose from 115.0 in 1960 to 131.0 in 1970. While this ratio is not quite as large as it is for the White population, the ratio for Negroes of all ages is over 110 as compared with only 105 for Whites, states Mr. Brotman.

_____. Facts and Figures on Older Americans. Washington, D. C.: Administration on Aging, No. 5, 1972, p. 3.

The writer surmises that the first counts from the 1970 census enumeration show a total of 22.7 million Blacks of all ages or 11.27% of the total population, an increase of about 3.8 million since 1960 when the figure was 18.9 million or 10.5% of the total population. As a result of lower life expectancy than is true for Whites, however, the Black aged in 1970 came to 1.6 million or only 7.8% of all of the aged. This was still an improvement over 1960 when the 1.2 million Black aged represented only 7.1% of all of the older persons in the United States. Stated another way, only 6.9% of the total Black population is aged 65+ as compared with over 10% for the Whites, concludes the author.

_____. Facts and Figures on Older Americans: State
Trends, 1960-1970. Washington, D. C.: Administration on Aging, No. 6, 1974, pp. 4-5.

The author states that between 1960 and 1970 the number of Negroes 65 years of age and older grew faster
than the total Negro population. This age group increased from 1.2 million in 1960 to 1.6 million in
1970. Since this was a higher rate of growth than
that of the total Negro population, the 65+ Negroes
accounted for 6.9% of the total Negro population as
compared to 6.2% in 1960. Although 6.9% is the national average for the aged Negro population, the
trend in numbers and in proportion of this population
varied considerably among the States, states the writer. He also points out that in terms of rates of
change between 1960 and 1970, six states had substantial growth of 100 percent (doubling) or over in
their aged Negro population--North Dakota 175.0%,
Alaska 142.2%, Nevada 122.7%, Hawaii 108.8%, Maine
107.3%, and Wisconsin 104.2%. These increases, however, were over very low numbers in 1960, ranging
from a low of 8 to a high of 2,051. In 1970, no
state had exactly the same percentage of aged Negroes as the national average, 6.9%. There were 16
states with larger proportions than the national average. The author concludes that at the lower end of
the distribution, 35 states had a smaller percentage
of aged Negroes than the national average. Eight of
these states were within one percentage point lower
than the national average (5.9-6.8). Thirteen states
were within two percentage points (4.9-5.8), and
seven within three points (3.9-4.8). Seven more
states were between four and six percentage points below the national average.

Hall, Gertrude and Geneva Mathiasen, Editors. Guide To
Development of Protective Services For Older People.
Springfield, Ill.: Charles C. Thomas Publishers,
1973.

The editors point out that in Houston and Philadelphia
a higher proportion of Negroes received protective
services than their ratio in the communities. In
Houston, 25.6 percent of the protective service clients were Negroes as compared with 16 percent Negro
population in the community. In Philadelphia, the
respective figures were 25 percent and 17 percent; in
San Diego, 11 percent and 3 percent.

Levitan, Sar A., William B. Johnston and Robert Taggart.
Still a Dream: The Changing Status of Blacks Since
1960. Cambridge: Harvard University Press, 1975.

The authors point out that overall, Blacks represented nearly one in ten Old Age Survivors and Disability

(Levitan, Sar A., William B. Johnston and Robert
Taggart)

Insurance (OASDI) recipients in 1971. Because Blacks
have shorter life expectancy, they accounted for only
7.5 percent of all retired workers receiving benefits,
which was nearly equivalent to their 7.9 percent share
of the elderly population (age sixty-two and over).
Under the survivors' segments, 7.7 percent of widows
receiving benefits were Black. The writers state that
Black life expectancies are considerably shorter than
Whites, meaning that Blacks are paying into a system
which is less likely to benefit them in later years.
They concluded that one approach which could correct
some of these problems would be to supplement payroll
taxes which contributed from general revenue.

McCann, Charles W. Long Beach Senior Citizens Survey.
Long Beach, Calif.: Community Welfare Council, 1955.

The author points out that in 1955 less than 1% of
Blacks lived in Long Beach that were 65 years old or
older. This was in contrast to the State of California as a whole where Blacks constituted 6% of the
population. Since the beginning of World War II,
Blacks have been coming to Long Beach in increasing
numbers. Drawn by work opportunities, they represented a relatively younger age group.

Rowan, Carl T. Just Between Us Blacks. New York: Random
House, 1974.

Section 65 discusses the Black Aged. The writer declares that about 1.6 million Black Americans are
sixty-five years and over. More than half of them
still live in the South, although the largest single
concentration is in New York City. Rowan argues that
we should find ways to give property-tax relief to the
elderly. He concludes that another way to aid older
men and women is to find some kind of work for them.
This would provide extra income, and it would furnish
a big psychological boost, letting them knew they
still belong and are useful.

State of New Jersey. New Jersey Old Age Assistance Report,
1937-1941. Trenton, N.J.: Department of Institutions
and Agencies, 1942.

The proportion of Black cases among recipients of old
age assistance was higher in 1938 than in 1937. According to the 1930 federal census 2.6 percent of the
population 65 years of age and over in New Jersey were
Black. In 1935 the proportion of Blacks on old age
assistance rolls was 9.4. The percentage had increased
to 10.1 in 1937, and in June, 1938 reached 10.9 percent. Thirteen percent of applications granted during

(State of New Jersey)

the year were those of Blacks. The increasing proportion of Blacks on old age assistance takes on significance when the problems peculiar to the group, particularly the Black's extreme need for adequate housing,
are borne in mind. The problem is one of first importance in at least two counties where almost one-third
of the entire case load is Black, according to the
report.

5. BLACK AGED AND MENTAL HEALTH

Butler, Robert N. and Myrna I. Lewis. Aging and Mental
    Health: Positive Psychological Approaches. St. Louis,
    Mo.: C. V. Mosby Co., 1973.

There is one section that discusses the Black Elderly.
The authors point out that since Black older people
die at a younger age, they may never become eligible
for retirement benefits even if they have them. It
was also pointed out that old people of all races
make up only 4% to 5% of community mental health clientele, so one can see that only a small fraction of
the total are Black. Also less than 3% of nursing
homes and homes for the aged residents are Black, according to the authors. The authors argue that the
Black church has proved to be a stabilizing force,
providing the elderly with social participation, prestige, and power in the internal life created by pa-
rishioners.

6. BLACK AGED AND OLD FOLKS' HOMES

DuBois, W. E. Burghardt and Augustus Granville Dill.
    Morals and Manners Among Negro Americans. Atlanta:
    Atlanta University Press, 1914.

Chapter Eleven discusses "Caring For Old People." The
authors declare that from early times Blacks in the
United States have established old folks' homes and
have now (1914) perhaps a hundred such homes throughout the land. They sent out questionnaires to twenty-
five states concerning the care of the Black aged.
The writers found that the Black elderly were being
provided for by relatives, friends or some charitable
institutions. In most cases they were receiving adequate care.

DuBois, W. E. B. Efforts For Social Betterment Among
    Negro Americans. Atlanta, Ga.: Atlanta University
    Press, 1909.

Section 11 in this book is devoted to "Old Folks'
Homes." The writer discusses the various homes for
the Black aged all over the United States from the

(DuBois, W. E. B.)

first one established in 1864 in Philadelphia to the
latest one established in 1907 in Detroit. He mentioned 61 Black Old Folks' Homes. Dr. DuBois points
out the breaking up of families in slavery by SALE and
during the war and Reconstruction times, greatly ag-
gravated the suffering of the old, while the loosened
family ties, due to the slave system, left in post-
bellum times numbers of neglected old folk. The author concludes, however, that even loose family ties
were not able to overcome the native African rever-
ence for parents, and before the war began Old Folks'
Homes for Negroes had begun to be established, some
by Negroes themselves, others by their friends.

Home For Aged Colored Women. <u>Forty-Seventh Annual Report
Of The Directors Of The Home For Aged Colored Women</u>.
Boston: Home For Aged Colored Women, 1907.

It was pointed out that outside relief is given to
forty aged and infirm colored women, in sums from
two dollars to six dollars per month, amounting in
all to one hundred and seventy-two dollars per month.
The number of inmates is limited to twenty, and applicants for admission must be sixty years old or over,
except in special cases of illness or infirmity. The
report goes on to state that the number of outside
beneficiaries has steadily increased, so that forty
women are now receiving sums of three to six dollars
a month, a total of one hundred and seventy-two being
paid out every month. It is the intention of the
directors to make this work as comprehensive as possible, and the Committee on Admissions has taken it
diligently in hand, conferring with other agencies
and individuals, and personally investigating all applications. They also visit those who already receive an allowance, to make sure that it is proving
sufficient and being wisely spent, and to recommend
an increase when advancing age and infirmity render
it necessary. There are many pathetic cases where
relatives or friends are making a hard struggle to
support these aged and feeble women, or a neighbor,
on whom there is no claim, has taken one in for chari-
ty's sake, and a small addition to the family income
eases the strain and makes better care possible.
There are also women who have supported themselves
all their lives, and cannot bear to sit down quietly
in a Home as long as they can do a little work outside, and this monthly allowance helps them to maintain their independence. The Home stands ready as a
refuge for all when outside resources fail. In it
they find rest and warmth, good food and care, a little work for those who are able, and an atmosphere of
cheerfulness and good-will which is rarely equaled
elsewhere. Matron and help, inmates and directors,

(Home For Aged Colored Women)

feel the mutual helpfulness and dependence on each
other of a real family, while everyone is free to fol-
low her own way provided they do not interfere with
the safety or comfort of others.

National Council on Aging. The Golden Years--A Tarnished
Myth. New York: National Council on Aging, 1970.

It was pointed out that while nursing homes certified
by Medicare are believed to be quantitatively better
than homes which cannot meet Medicare requirements,
the aged poor, who are usually Black, do not always
take advantage of the Medicare facilities.

7. BLACKS AND MINORITY AGED

Butler, Robert N. Why Survive? Being Old in America.
New York: Harper & Row, 1975.

The author looks to more sensitive treatment of minority aged at the point of service provision as a factor
that could be effective in increasing their utilization of social services. Noting that minority groups
are extremely poorly represented in the service professions as doctors, nurses, and social workers, Butler suggests that those providing services to minority aged "should have the assistance of interpreters
and training with respect to language and culture when
this is appropriate. The service provider must understand the differing patterns of behavior that affect
the giving and receiving of service."

Cohen, Elias. Minority Aged in America. Ann Arbor: Institute of Gerontology, University of Michigan, 1972.

The author points out that where the more affluent
elderly have received benefits almost automatically,
the poor and the minority elderly must contend with a
bewildering mixture of programs and policies which often bear little relationship to their real or perceived needs.

Weeks, Herbert A. and Benjamin J. Darsky. The Urban Aged:
Race and Medical Care. Ann Arbor: University of
Michigan, School of Public Health, 1968.

The writers point out that the urban Black aged receive less medical care than other ethnic groups.
The medical facilities are not always easily accessible to the Black elderly. Therefore they are at a
great disadvantage when it comes to proper health care.

8. URBAN BLACK AGED

Drake, St. Clair and Horace R. Cayton. Black Metropolis:
A Study of Negro Life In A Northern City (Chicago).
New York: Harcourt, Brace and Co., 1945.

Various aged Black residents of Chicago recall the
"good" old days in that city. They were referring to
the 1900-1940s. Many state that things were relatively "good" for Blacks before a large number of
Blacks migrated from the South to that Northern city.

Frazier, E. Franklin. The Negro Family in Chicago. Chicago: University of Chicago Press, 1932.

Several "old" Black residents of Chicago viewed with
alarm the influx of the ignorant masses from the South
migrating to Chicago. They saw their neighborhoods
deteriorating and met racial barriers where none had
existed before. To them, the migrants constituted a
threat to the standards of behavior which they had
safeguarded as a heritage. The aged Blacks even
formed such clubs as "The Old Settlers Club" in order
to separate themselves from those "hordes of barbari-
ans," concludes Dr. Frazier.

9. COMPARATIVE BLACK AND WHITE AGED

Butler, Robert N. Why Survive? Being Old in America.
New York: Harper & Row, 1975.

Various references are made to the Black aged throughout the book. The author declares in absolute numbers more Whites than Blacks are elderly poor (85
percent of the total elderly poor are White, 15 percent Black). Black poverty, however, is more profound
than White poverty. The percentage of aged Blacks
living in poverty is twice that of aged Whites. For-
ty-seven percent of all aged Black females have incomes under $1,000. In rural areas two out of three
aged Blacks fall below the poverty line. Furthermore,
elderly Blacks tend to have more people dependent on
them than do the White elderly. More elderly Black
people live with younger people than do White elderly;
28 percent of them live in families with a young head
of household compared to 8.9 percent for all elderly,
regardless of race. There are many reasons why a larger percentage of Black elderly live with their children: the importance of the role of grandmother because the mother works or is away; the need for the
sharing of income within a family, including the older person's Social Security and public assistance payments; and the respect and sense of responsibility,
said to exist more strongly in Black households, in
caring for and protecting one's parents, particularly
the aged mother. The author continues to surmise that

(Butler, Robert N.)

those older Blacks who do not live with relatives are
in a much more disadvantaged economic situation: 75
percent of all elderly Blacks living alone fall below
the poverty line, and Project FIND reported that of
Black widows an amazing 85 percent were living in poverty, with another 5 percent on the borderline.
These are depressing facts indeed for an affluent society.   The impacts of racism upon aging are reflected
in life expectancies at time of birth, which in turn
affect retirement benefits.   The average life expectancy of Black males has actually declined by a year
over the 1960-70 decade.   Among males, non-White death
rates were higher than those of Whites through age 76,
with a reversal occurring beyond that age.   Non-White
female death rates were higher than White female
death rates through age 77.   Dr. Butler concludes that
there is a need to reflect differences in racial life
expectancies by lowering the minimum age-eligibility
requirements for other pensions as well, since few
elderly Blacks live long enough to collect benefits,
according to the writer.

Grier, William H. and Price M. Cobbs.   Black Rage. New
York: Basic Books, 1968.

Various references are made throughout the book to
aged Blacks.   The writers point out how young and old
Blacks resent White people.   Some Blacks express their
resentfulness openly and others suppress it.   One
example in this work, an eighty-seven year old Black
woman still recalls how her mother spoke up for her
to her White employer in the South during slavery.

Hoffman, Adeline M.   The Daily Needs and Interests of
Older People.   Springfield, Ill.:   Charles C. Thomas,
Publisher, 1970.

The writer asserts that one might hypothesize that the
Black aged have fewer problems than Whites in accommo-
dating the normative demands of the kin group because
of previous experience and identification within it.
The author concludes that the service orientation is
more pronounced among the Black subculture, especially the lower class and undoubtedly there are height-
ened reciprocal activities among its members and a
useful service role for the aged Black.

Kalish, Richard A.   Late Adulthood: Perspectives on Human
Development.   Monterey, Calif.:   Brooks/Cole Publishing Co., 1975.

Various references are made to the Black aged throughout the book.   In most of the references the author

(Kalish, Richard A.)

compares them with other minority ethnic groups as well as with the White aged. He contends that the Black aged have led a doubly difficult life. First, they are victimized by overt or covert prejudice and discrimination or by their lack of language skills, vocational training, and opportunity. Second, they now find themselves under attack for not having been aggressive enough at an earlier age against these injustices or for not being able to alter their values sufficiently in their later years. Kalish concludes, however, that there is an increasing appreciation of the plight of the general community.

Kent, Donald P. and Carl Hirsch, et al. <u>Needs and Use of Services Among Negro and White Aged</u>. Vol. I. University Park, Pa.: Pennsylvania State University, July, 1971.

The writers state differentials in income level, with the oldest Black respondents suffering greatest financial deprivation, occurred at levels below those determined to be minimal for adequate maintenance among the sample as a whole. Disparities that do occur on a racial basis were found to exist only between Blacks and Whites residing with family members who may be seen to serve as a buffer between the Black aged and the most severe consequences of such limited financial resources. The author found that a greater proportion of Black respondents than White were working, even if retired, in order to maintain their present income levels. While more Blacks than Whites were dependent on welfare allotments for income maintenance, this pattern seems to result from lesser degrees of eligibility among Blacks for both private and government pension programs based on employment in earlier years, according to the authors. Through the authors' general knowledge of rampant discrimination against Blacks in the crucial employment area, they saw the results of lessened economic security when old age is reached among Blacks compared to Whites even in a group selected from areas of low socio-economic status in a city. Differences between the racial groups were also found in the area of informal social interaction. However, while Black respondents were found to have fewer living children than Whites, the total ability for dependence within the social networks of the respondents was not uniformly weighted in favor of the White aged in this sample. Rather, state Kent and Hirsch, differences by age are often most notable with older respondents in both race groups faring less well. In residential situations they found Black respondents more often subject to poor housing conditions than Whites. White respondents are more often found to be the owners of their

(Kent, Donald P. and Carl Hirsch, et al.)

residences or living in homes that are owned by a member of the household. The authors conclude that the
research results reported may be shown to call for
greater attention to poor aged community residents,
both Black and White, by government and voluntary
agencies whose defined goals include supports for an
improved quality of life among urban residents. This
study was done in the Philadelphia Model Cities area.

_____. Health Conditions, Social Adjustment, and Uti-
lization of Community Resources Among Negro and White
Aged. Vol. II. University Park, Pa.: Pennsylvania
State University, October, 1972.

The title tells what this work is about. The authors
state that in all areas, health conditions, utilization of community resources, housing, financial aid
counseling, employment services, transportation, one
finds that the Black aged is at the bottom of the
ladder. This work is a follow-up of Vol. I by the
same authors. They conclude that it would be self
deluding to imagine that the earlier reporting (Vol.
I) of these findings would have significantly contributed to be a change of conditions in the lives of
the sampled population or in the activities of the
agencies delegated by society to work with the aged.
On the other hand, continue the authors, it is also
disappointing to appreciate that little change has
occurred within these two spheres in the time that
has passed since fieldwork began. This study was
done in the Philadelphia Model Cities area.

Kivi, Ronald E., et al., Editors. Michigan Aging Citizens:
Characteristics, Opinions, and Service Utilization
Patterns. Ann Arbor, Michigan: Institute of Gerontology, University of Michigan-Wayne State University,
1975.

Various references are made throughout the book to the
Black aged. The elderly Blacks live in Detroit and
other cities, and as a group, they have lower incomes
than White older people. Black aging citizens also
had less formal education than White ones. The editors surmise that there were no differences between
Black and White older people in Detroit in their responses to: (a) desire to move; (b) satisfaction with
the neighborhood as a place to live; (c) satisfaction
with general appearance of neighborhood; (d) satisfaction with neighborhood police protection; and (e)
satisfaction with the safety of the place where they
lived. More elderly Blacks than elderly Whites had
problems getting enough medical care. More Black aged
than older Whites cited television as their primary
source of community information.

Manard, Barbara Bolling, et al. Old-Age Institutions.
    Lexington, Mass.: Lexington Books, 1975.

    The author points out that the states with the larg-
    est non-White elderly populations are Southern. The
    seventeen states in which fewer than 3 percent of the
    elderly are non-White--Colorado, Connecticut, Florida,
    Massachusetts, Minnesota, Montana, Nebraska, New Hamp-
    shire, North Dakota, Oregon, Rhode Island, South Da-
    kota, Utah, Vermont, Washington, Wisconsin, and Wyom-
    ing--are predominantly north central and eastern. Two
    urban northeastern states, Massachusetts and Rhode Is-
    land, have elderly populations that are less than 2
    percent Black; in New York and New Jersey, the pro-
    portion is about 6 percent. Thus, the distribution
    of the states with respect to the proportion of the
    elderly population that is non-White closely mirrors
    the distribution along other dimensions we have found
    to be associated with low rates of institutionaliza-
    tion, state the authors. This fact probably contri-
    butes to the underrepresentation of Blacks in the to-
    tal Old-Age Institutions (OAI) population: Blacks
    are less likely than Whites, nationally, to be in OAI
    because Blacks, by and large, live in states where
    old people in general are less likely to be in OAI.
    Looking at Virginia, Blacks comprise 18 percent of
    the elderly population and 12 percent of the elderly
    population in OAI. In Virginia, elderly blacks are
    about as likely as elderly Whites to live in extra-
    familial situations, declare the writers. The propor-
    tions are 24 and 26 percent respectively. Since
    Blacks in Virginia are proportionately more likely
    than Whites to be in institutions other than OAI,
    when we group together the elderly populations in all
    types of institutions, we find little difference be-
    tween Blacks and Whites, conclude the authors. In
    Virginia, 4.5 percent of the elderly Whites and 4.4
    percent of the elderly Blacks are in institutions and
    group quarters. A similar situation occurs in Mass-
    achusetts, which has both a high proportion of its
    elderly in OAI and a low proportion of non-Whites gen-
    erally. Almost 2 percent (1.9) of the Massachusetts
    elderly population is Black, and 1.7 percent of the
    elderly OAI population is Black, according to the
    authors.

Smith, Bert Kruger. Aging in America. Boston: Beacon,
    1973.

    Part of Chapter Three is devoted to "Problems of Race
    and Poverty." The author asserts that almost one
    half of all the older Blacks are living below the pov-
    erty level. He also argues that with poverty came
    the ragged companions of poor housing and poor health.
    Life expectancy is much lower for Blacks than for
    Whites. The author concludes that although the Black

(Smith, Bert Kruger)

aged do not use the medical services as frequently as
Whites do, they have more intense illnesses, resulting in significantly more bed-disability days than
Whites of similar ages. The compound problems of age
and poverty and minority status, argues Smith, make
older years a constant hardship for many Americans.

10.   BLACK AGED AND THE BLACK CHURCH

Walls, William J. The African Methodist Epsicopal Zion
   Church: Reality of The Black Church. Charlotte,
   N. C.: A. M. E. Zion Publishing House, 1974.

Chapter 27 is entitled "Concern for Aged Ministers,
Widows and Children." As early as 1848, the A. M. E.
Zion Church provided for worn out (Aged) ministers.
In 1896 the General Conference organized a "Committee
on Worn-Out-Preachers." The church felt a responsibility to its aged ministers. The by-laws of the
church said that "if a minister is permanently in-
capacitated by reason of sickness or accident he is
eligible for retirement and pension."

11.   BLACK AGED AND MINORITY AGED

Barrow, Georgia M. and Patricia A. Smith. Aging, Ageism
   and Society. With Cartoons by Bulbul. St. Paul,
   Minn.: West Publishing Co., 1979.

Chapter 13 is devoted to "The Minority Aged." The
authors rely on data from previous printed works by
other writers for his material on the "Black Aged."
The writers conclude that Blacks are the largest
group of the aged minorities followed by Hispanics,
American Indians, and Asian Americans. According to
the authors, the numbers of persons do not reflect,
however, the variety in these groups in terms of
races, cultures, languages, socioeconomic status, and
historical or traditional attitudes and beliefs.
They also point out that upgrading the status of the
minority elderly requires recognition of the various
factors that prevent them from utilizing services followed by the establishment of outreach programs designed to overcome them.

Hess, Beth B., Editor. Growing Old in America. New Bruns-
   wick, N. J.: Transaction Books, 1976.

Several articles on the Black Aged in this collection
are reprinted from previous published works. There
are, however, several references to the Black aged
that present a different viewpoint. The editor in
her "introduction" declares "while it may be a facile
truism to say to be black and to be old in America

(Hess, Beth B.)

is a double yoke of oppression, the precise ways in
which race and age interact to influence one's treatment at the hands of functionaries (and well-meaning
sociologists), the allocation of scarce resources, or
access to opportunities for self-fulfillment are very
subtle indeed." Other articles in this book also al-
lude to the Black aged.

12. BLACK AGED AND OLD FOLKS' HOMES

Rebeck, Ann H. A Study Of The Developments in Programs For
The Care Of The Aged: With Emphasis on New York
State and New York City. New York: New York State
Department of Social Welfare, May 1, 1943.

In 1941 there were 73 private homes for the aged in
and around the metropolitan area serving residents
from New York City. Of that number, there were only
three (3) for the Blacks; two for Black women and one
for men and women. About six homes cared for both
Blacks and Whites. The writer concludes that although
there were long waiting lists for all homes, the need
for facilities for Blacks was the most acute. The
author also gives an example of a small home for
Black women.

4.

DISSERTATIONS
AND THESES

1. URBAN BLACK AGED

Beard, Virginia Harrison. "A Study of Aging Among A Successful, Urban Black Population." Unpublished Doctoral Dissertation, St. Louis University, 1976.

In this investigation an effort was made to identify some distinguishing characteristics more or less common to successful Black aged persons. The areas of investigation were life satisfaction, adjustment, the person's self perception of being Black in a predominantly White society. The group was identified by the criteria: 1. Education, at least a high school graduate, 2. Income, more than $3999 annually of a single aged person, 3. Health, reported to be in fair to excellent health, with no more than one chronic illness. Data was gathered by an extensive questionnaire including the Life Satisfaction Scale Index Z (LISZ), the Stages of Black Awareness Scale, and several questions constructed for use in this study to measure adjustment and change with age. Subjects were selected at random from rosters of Black organizations in St. Louis City and County and on recommendation of community people. The sample was 100 men and women ranging in age from 34 to 91 years, however, only six were below age 50. Conclusions indicated that successful Black aged, very much alike in certain socioeconomic ways, still appeared quite heterogeneous in terms of life satisfaction, Black self perception and by other variables. The researcher recommended that more studies of a descriptive and exploratory nature be done using larger numbers of subjects of successful Black aged and for other sub-groups in order to provide more information and to identify predictor variables. It was also recommended that the exclusion of Blacks from important aging studies should only be done when it can be determined and validated that race is an extraneous variable for the researching of a particular construct.

Dancy, Joseph J. "Religiosity and Social-Psychological Adjustment Among The Black Urban Elderly." Unpublished Doctoral Dissertation, University of Michigan, 1978.

This study addresses itself to two universal phenomena, aging and religion in an examination of the relationship of religion to the socio-psychological adjustment of the urban Black elderly. The data for this study is taken from an earlier study conducted by Gary T. Marx of the University of California which originally focused on anti-semitism in the United States. The total sample of that study included 1,119 Black metropolitan residents of which 182 persons were age 60 and over. The latter group constitutes the respondents in this present study. These data include six questions which could serve as measures of religiosity. These questions related to (1) belief in God, (2) Jesus as Savior, (3) importance of religiosity, (4) life beyond death, (5) existence of the devil, and (6) attendance at worship services. The primary mode of examining the relationship between religiosity and socio-psychological adjustment was through use of cross-tabulations and correlations. In an effort to determine the extent to which this relationship could be explained by the demographic variables, multi-variate tables, partial correlations, and multiple regression were utilized. According to the author, the results indicated that those factors which most decidedly separated those Black elderly who measured high in religiosity from those who measured low in religiosity were: income, being raised on a farm, sex, educational level, and number of years at present residence. The Black elderly, overall, showed a high level of religiosity by responding quite strongly to the extreme favorable position of the six religiosity items. When the six religiosity items were considered by sex, females showed a higher response to these items than the males on every item. Data also revealed that persons of lower socioeconomic status are more religious than those of higher socioeconomic status. The writer concludes that with regard to adjustment, there appeared to be little overall difference in the adjustment of older Black urban males when compared with older Black urban females. However, class differences were major factors in adjustment with the higher class group of older Blacks appearing better adjusted than the lower class group as measured by the twelve items of adjustment.

Dhaliwal, Sher Singh. "A Sociological Description and Analysis of A Non-Random Sample of Low-Income, Washington, D. C., Aged Negroes." Unpublished Master's Thesis, Howard University, 1967.

(Dhaliwal, Sher Singh)

The author describes selected social characteristics
of an elderly group living in a low-income area of
Washington, D. C. The charactersitics studied were
living arrangements and conditions, economic status,
social and leisure time activities, religious and civ-
ic activities, and attitudes toward themselves, death,
living arrangements and programs for the aged.

Lambing, Mary L. "A Study of Retired Older Negroes in an
    Urban Setting." Unpublished Doctoral Dissertation,
    University of Florida, 1969.

The purpose of this study was to investigate the life-
style of American Blacks retiring from the professions, from stable blue-collar work, and from the service occupations, domestic work, and common labor.
Data were obtained from interviews of 101 retired
Blacks in Alachus County, Florida. About one-third
of the interviews were carried out by non-Whites. Because social class membership has repeatedly been
found to be an important determinant of behavior, this
factor was emphasized throughout the study. The A. B.
Hollingshead Two-Factor Index of Social Position was
used to ascertain social status of respondents. Thirteen former professionals were interviewed, which constituted a local availability sample made up primarily
of school teachers. There were only 15 retirees from
blue-collar occupations who could be included in the
study. A representative sample of 73 people drawn
from the rolls of the Department of Public Welfare had
been in service occupations, domestic work, and common labor. Some of the latter group were also recipients of social security benefits. Retired Blacks
had an average of 3.02 living children. Of those with
living children, 25% lived in the same household with
a child and 52% had at least one child living in the
same town. Fifty-six percent saw their children weekly or more often. Indications were that these Blacks
had much closer relationships with siblings than retired people in studies made with White subjects. Mutual assistance patterns were similar to those found
in earlier gerontological research. When a study of
active roles was made, these Blacks did not show evidence of disengagement after the age of 65. Church
and church-related activities represented the greatest
proportion of voluntary association memberships. More
women than men belonged to organizations. Some decrease in activity was seen with advancing age, but
social class, level of education, and income were
stronger determinants of involvement. The author concludes that the evidence for disengagement was not
strong. Elderly Blacks tended to carry on the activities and interaction patterns they had prior to retirement and when they disengaged it was because they

(Lambing, Mary L.)

were forced to do so when their income was lowered.

Sauer, William J. "Morale of The Urban Aged: A Regression Analysis By Race." Unpublished Doctoral Dissertation, University of Minnesota, 1975.

Past research in the field of social gerontology has paid little concern to morale of aged Blacks. The purpose of this research was to develop a model, based primarily on previous research on aged White samples, and examine the degree to which the predictors of morale were isomorphic for aged Whites and aged Blacks. A search of the literature revealed that such a model would consist of the following variables: Age, sex, race, education, occupation, income, marital status, health, participation in voluntary associations, interaction with relatives, friends and neighbors. Hypotheses were formulated linking each of these independent variables to morale (the Lawton PGC scale was used in this research) and testing the hypothesis for both Blacks and Whites. The data consisted of a random sample of low income aged Blacks and Whites in Philadelphia and were collected by the late Donald P. Kent as part of the Aged Services Project he was directing. The sample consisted of 936 elderly, 722 of which were Black and 214 of which were White. All respondents were 65 years of age or older. The data were analyzed using regression analysis. Rather than use statistical significance as the major criterion for testing the hypotheses it was decided to use standardized beta coefficients of ±.15 to offset the large sample size. The author argues that the results of the analyses indicated for Blacks the only two significant predictors of morale were health and participation in solitary activities, with the former being the most important. For Whites, in addition to health and solitary activities, interaction with family and sex were also found to be significant. Unlike Blacks, however, solitary activities were the most important followed by health, with sex and family interaction being of lesser importance. It was concluded that for these data the predictors are not isomorphic between races; further work is needed using more heterogeneous samples to demonstrate the differences the proposed model suggests exist between races. Finally, the implications of this research to current gerontological research are discussed.

Smith, Alicia D. "Life Satisfaction and Activity Preference Among Black Inner City Center Participants: An Exploratory Study." Unpublished Doctoral Dissertation, University of Massachusetts, 1978.

The purpose of this investigation was to identify

(Smith, Alicia D.)

Black senior center participants who reside in a
northeastern urban community, and to determine if
there is a relationship between individual preferences
for particular learning activities and those living
conditions which account for life satisfaction. In
addition, the study was intended to investigate the
elderly's perceptions of "survival" or coping needs.
The results indicate that (1) the population of Black
senior center participants tend to be as diverse as
the general population, (2) health, length of residency and age are significant correlates of life satisfaction, (3) length of residence is the single best
predictor of life satisfaction, and (4) participants
prefer activities which are personal and health related. The importance of the leisure and social atmosphere at the centers in attracting participants and
the possibility that survival skills perceptions may
be a result of the interaction between reality and
attitudes as defined by life and cultural experiences,
are emerging issues. It is concluded that, for this
population, aging adjustment means engaging in and enlarging upon social interactions and experiences rather than disengaging.

Williams, Lois L. "Analysis of Social and Community Needs
    of Black Senior Citizens in Inner City Detroit." Un-
    published Doctoral Dissertation, University of Michi-
    gan, 1977.

    The purpose of this study was to make available some
    information concerning the complex needs of the Black
    senior citizen and to identify supportive services
    designed to enhance the capacity of this elderly pop-
    ulation to improve its quality of life. The results
    indicated that the majority of the Black senior citi-
    zens were found to be satisfied with their living con-
    ditions despite a multitude of seemingly negative
    characteristics such as: 1) Substandard housing fa-
    cilities located in the midst of an urban area, 2)
    Presence of an unusually high crime rate, 3) A
    relatively low socio-economic status, 4) Apparent
    psychological conditions of resignation, 5) A sense
    of complacency with respect to those areas over which
    they felt they had no control. The results and impli-
    cations of the study suggest future research in the
    following areas: 1) A study to delineate the pecu-
    liar problems attendant to the aging Black urban poor
    in America as contrasted to those common to other
    urban populations, 2) A study to determine the needs
    of Black senior citizens living in their own home
    sites as opposed to those living in public facilities,
    3) A comparative study of the success of social ser-
    vice agencies in delivering identical basic social
    services to (a) senior citizens in public high-rise

(Williams, Lois L.)

housing as contrasted to (b) senior citizens in their
own home sites.

2. RURAL AGED BLACK

Ball, Mercedes Elizabeth. "Comparison of Characteristics
    of Aged Negroes In Two Counties." Unpublished Mas-
    ter's Thesis, Howard University, 1967.

This study was done to find selected characteristics
of an elderly group of rural and urban Blacks to com-
pare patterns of aging in Dodge and Chatham counties
in Georgia. The characteristics included housing,
family and friendship relationships, leisure and recreation, religious and social activities, use of local
programs and facilities, health, education, and economic status.

Davis, Abraham, Jr. "Selected Characteristic Patterns of A
    Southern Aged Rural Negro Population." Unpublished
    Master's Thesis, Howard University, 1966.

This is a descriptive survey of selected social characteristics of the aged, rural Blacks in Macon County,
Alabama. The author discusses such characteristics
as living conditions, family and friendship relationships, leisure time and religious activities, attitudes toward desired residential patterns, problems
and death, awareness and use of facilities for the
aged and health problems.

3. BLACK AGED AND HOUSING

Anderson, Peggye D. "The Black Aged: Dispositions Toward
    Seeking Age Concentrated Housing in a Small Town."
    Unpublished Doctoral Dissertation, Northwestern Uni-
    versity, 1975.

This work is an exploratory study in which the author
searched for elderly Blacks' attitudes toward seeking
aged concentrated housing as well as factors that influence their desire to seek this style of living.
The study includes 208 Black elderly people sixty-five
years and older. The setting in which the study was
conducted is Tuskegee, Alabama. The lives and lifestyles of the Black elderly people in the study do not
vary much from the general aged population. Their
level of education, marital and health status reflect
the typical aged person. Thus, the people in this
study have an average of eight years of schooling.
The majority of the females are widowed and the majority of the males are married. Most of the people are
in good to fair health. The author also found that
even though some variables do not help explain why

(Anderson, Peggye D.)

aged Blacks may seek age concentrated housing; nevertheless, they provide interesting insight into the
lives and lifestyles of Black elderly people. Such
variables that help us understand more about elderly
Black people's lives, but not help explain why the elderly would seek age concentrated housing, include:
family relations, sex, age and age identification.

Hawkins, Brin D. "A Comparative Study of the Social Par-
    ticipation of The Black Elderly Residing in Public
    Housing in Two Communities: The Inner City and the
    Suburbs." Unpublished Doctoral Dissertation, Brandeis
    University, 1976.

This study was based on a sample of 145 elderly Black
men and women residing in two public housing projects
in the Washington, D. C. area. The Claridge project
is located in an inner city, high crime, high density,
predominantly Black census tract. The Regency is located in a low crime, low density, predominantly
White suburban fringe census tract. The basic premise
of this study is that social participation can serve
as a mediating function between the role loss experienced in the later years and morale, because it provides supports to the individual's role identities
which are prerequisites for a positive self-concept.
A major factor influencing social participation is the
residential environment, which may inhibit or facili-
tate social interaction. Personal characteristics
were also considered as they influence social participation in old age; i.e., sex, age, marital status, education, income, and relocation experience. The findings of this study support the adaptability of older
persons, particularly the ability of the Black elderly
to adjust to a new and unfamiliar residential environment. The findings further indicate a higher level of
interaction in clubs or organized activity in a
pleasant and safe community where opportunities for
social interaction are available. The above findings
in concert with the positive relationship found between social participation and morale, serve as the
basis for the policy implications and recommendations
contained in this study.

Stretch, John J. "The Development and Testing of a Theore-
    tical Formulation That Aged Negroes With Differences
    in Community Security Are Different in Coping Reac-
    tions." Unpublished Doctoral Dissertation, Tulane
    University, 1967.

This study conceptualized and tested a beginning
theory developed by the author from social-psychological and neo-psychoanalytic sources, that there are
differences in coping reactions between two popula-

(Stretch, John J.)

tions of aged Blacks who have differences in community security. The sample used was seventy-two
Blacks, predominantly sixty years old and above, not
living with spouse, and meeting eligibility requirements for residence in the William Guste public housing apartment. The findings in general, confirmed
the beginning theoretical formulation as conceptualized. No significant differences were found between
the Guste-Community group on nineteen extraneous variables thought to influence coping. Significant differences in the predicted direction for the Low Security sample on six of these variables were found
between the High-Low Security group. Differences in
the six community security scores were in the predicted direction of higher scores for the Guste Homes
sample than for the Community sample, with two scores,
total community security and self-fulfillment, significant beyond the five percent level. Of the two empirical indicators of community security, larger sample differences in coping reaction scores were found
between the High-Low Security group than between the
Guste-Community group. Most differences in coping
reaction scores, nineteen out of twenty-four were in
the predicted direction, and in the High-Low Security
group eight were significant, concludes the writer.

Sugg, Michael L. "A Comparative Study of Morale and Activity Levels Among Lower Socio-Economic Elderly Residents Living in Age-Segregated vs. Age-Integrated
Housing Arrangements." Unpublished Doctoral Dissertation, University of Pittsburgh, 1975.

The central concern of this study is the theoretical
and policy implications related to what type of living arrangements are most suitable for elderly poor
persons. A comparative design was implemented utilizing the theoretical orientation of the so-called Activity theory and Disengagement theory while assessing
the activity and morale levels of age-segregated versus age-integrated living arrangements among a total
research population of 402 elderly poor obtained from
two social service agencies in Allegheny County, Pennsylvania. Three separate residential groups were compared: (1) Public housing, age-segregated elderly;
(2) Public housing, age-integrated elderly; (3) Private housing, age-integrated elderly. An activity
scale was utilized and morale levels were measured
by Havighurst's much used morale scale. The findings
indicated that both theories were rejected in relation to age-segregated elderly, but not entirely in
the case of private dwelling, age-integrated elderly.
Activity and morale scores regardless of health, age,
or other variables, were consistently higher for both
age-segregated and age-integrated elderly living in

(Sugg, Michael L.)

public housing arrangements. Private housing, age-in-tegrated elderly with satisfactory morale levels and low activity scores reflected a disengaged style of life. The overall findings, then, strongly support a policy of expanded development in public housing for the elderly in our society.

4. BLACK AGED WOMEN

Chapman, Sabrina Coffey. "A Social-Psychological Analysis of Morale In a Selected Population: Low-Income El-derly Black Females." Unpublished Doctoral Disser-tation, Pennsylvania State University, 1979.

This study concerned itself with the relationships existing between certain social-psychological varia-bles and morale in a select minority population, low-income elderly Black females, and also analyzes the differences in morale existing between the study pop-ulation and low-income elderly White females. It was reasoned that, although the low-income elderly Black female is in a precarious position of multiple jeo-pardy in the larger sociocultural milieu, her posi-tion within the Black community itself is a highly esteemed one. Historically, and of necessity, aged Black females have often, over their life-spans, ty-pically assumed both the instrumental role, that of providing the family's economic support, and the in-tegrative, expressive role, that of providing inter-generational family support. Accordingly, the theo-retical constructs of role continuity--role discon-tinuity and activity theory, as well as those of re-lative deprivation--relative gain and disengagement theory, were utilized as pertained to the research problem. It was found that no significant relation-ship could be established between race and morale. The fact that the difference in morale levels was not verifiable as statistically significant between low-income elderly Black females and low-income elderly White females seems to suggest that the life experi-ences of these two populations are more parallel than anticipated; and, that the similarities attendant to the experience of being old, poor and female are greater than the dissimilarities of that experience, regardless of race.

Hamlett, Margaret Lucylle. "An Exploratory Study of The Socio-Economic and Psychological Problems of Adjust-ment of 100 Aged and Retired Negro Women in Durham, North Carolina During 1959." Unpublished Master's Thesis, North Carolina College at Durham, 1959.

The author states that three-quarters of the women were reasonably well adjusted. According to Ms.

(Hamlett, Margaret Lucylle)

Hamlett an analysis of the data indicated that a greater proportion of the women had problems in the economic than in either the psychological or social areas. Most of the social activities they performed prior to old age were continued. It was also found that the factor of race was not a basis for the maladjustment of these women. She concludes that the generally accepted beliefs with reference to the problems of the aged are inadequate in many respects when applied to a selected sample of aged and retired women residing in Durham, North Carolina during 1959.

5.   BLACK AGED MEN

Adam, Antenor Joseph. "An Exploratory Study of The Relation of The Adjustment of 100 Aged Negro Men in Durham, North Carolina With Their Education, Health, and Work Status." Unpublished Master's Thesis, North Carolina College at Durham, 1961.

The writer found that the over-all adjustment levels of the subjects studied were, on the average, high. There was no difference between economic status and adjustment, and social status and adjustment. Adam found that there was no difference between psychological status and adjustment and economic status and adjustment. The highness of the mean scores of the social, economic, and psychological adjustment areas is accounted for in part by the selectivity of the group studied. Non-welfare status, which indicates a relative absence of poverty, was used as a reference point in the choice of subjects.

6.   BLACK AGED AND THE BLACK FAMILY

Yelder, Josephine E. "Generational Relationships in Black Families: Some Perceptions of Grandparents' Role." Unpublished Doctoral Dissertation, University of Southern California, 1975.

This study investigated themes and variations in the role of grandparents in Black families. The research involved a descriptive analysis of grandparenting and its relationship to other variables. A purposive sample of forty-one Black grandparents with a grandchild between the ages of four and five years was selected. The primary method of data collection was through interviews with these participants in their homes. Data were gathered during a three month period regarding demographic factors, perceptions of family relationships, grandparent role, child rearing opinions, and relationships outside the family. Three major working hypotheses guided this study: (1) the style of grandparenting will vary with the changing circum-

(Yelder, Josephine E.)

stances of grandparents, parents, and/or grandchildren; (2) generational relationships in Black families are a network of roles in which the grandparent
role is an acquired role that is in part influenced
by the significance of the role to the occupant; and
(3) the degree of comfort in being a grandparent will
be related to factors which influence what is perceived as normative in the performance of the grandparent role. The author concludes that the respondents ranged in age from 43-75 years and had 107 children, 248 grandchildren and 52 great grand-children.
Close family ties were indicated by most of the group.
Most of the respondents felt that child rearing practices should be flexible to fit the needs of the child.
Evidences of generation gaps tended not to include
those factors related to family solidarity, states the
author. Generally it was felt that a generation gap
existed between adjacent generations but not between
nonadjacent generations. Participants were involved
in a variety of activities outside the family.

7. RELIGION AND THE BLACK AGED

Gray, Cleo J. "Attitudes of Black Church Members Towards
   The Black Elderly As a Function of Denomination, Age,
   Sex, and Level of Education." Unpublished Doctoral
   Dissertation, Howard University, 1977.

As an initial empirical venture in the study of attitudes held--and thus communicated--by Blacks, this
study focuses only on the response of this population
to the aged Black. The study is further limited with
respect to age, sex, level of education and membership in a Black church, the major interacting institution in the life of the aged. Using a study sample
drawn from the total population of male and female
members of three different denominations and churches
(N=210), and employing Kogan's Attitude Toward Old
People Scale (a Likert-type scale of 17 matched posi-
tive-negative pairs), the following null hypotheses
were tested: (1) There is no significant difference
in the attitude of Black church members toward the
elderly as a function of denomination. (2) There is
no significant difference in the attitude of Black
church members toward the elderly as a function of
age. (3) There is no significant difference in the
attitude of Black church members toward the elderly
as a function of sex. (4) There is no significant
difference in the attitude of Black church members
toward the elderly as a function of level of education.
The writer concludes that as the data suggest that a
positive attitudinal climate exists in the Black
church and is thus communicated. Recommendations were
made to structure and implement programming and acti-

(Gray, Cleo J.)

vities which serve to enlarge the positive climate and
to mitigate against the propagation of negative attitudes toward the elderly.

8.   BLACK AGED AND LIFE SATISFACTION

Bailey, Shirley Barrett. "A Study of Selected Factors Re-
     lated To The Social Satisfaction of the Residents Of
     A Facility For Senior Citizens--The Roosevelt For
     Senior Citizens." Unpublished Master's Thesis, Howard
     University, 1975.

     The author looks at the factors related to the social
     satisfaction of residents of the Roosevelt for Senior
     Citizens. The study was done to find out if residents
     were satisfied with living conditions with friends and
     relatives, and if lower income residents were as
     pleased as higher income residents.

Harper, D. W., Jr. "Socialization For The Aged Status
     Among the Negro." Unpublished Master's Thesis, Lou-
     isiana State University at Baton Rouge, 1967.

     The author points out that the larger Black community
     should take more interest in the Black aged and should
     be more responsive to their needs. According to the
     writer the aged Black should have more contact with
     their own age group and to the larger Black community.

Peterson, John L. "Personality Effects of Self-Esteem,
     Need Motivation, and Locus of Control on The Life
     Satisfaction of Older Black Adults." Unpublished Doc-
     toral Dissertation, University of Michigan, 1974.

     The author points out that although the psychological
     effects of aging have begun to receive considerable
     attention among White adults, few studies have been
     concerned with these effects among other ethnic groups.
     If similar results could be found for different ethnic
     groups as that available for White samples, there
     would be greater support for theories concerned with
     personality effects of aging. This assumption prompt-
     ed the investigation of the influence of personality
     factors on life satisfaction among older Black adults.
     Specifically, the personality factors which were as-
     sumed to affect life satisfaction were: 1) self-es-
     teem; 2) need motivation: need achievement (n Ach),
     need affiliation (n Aff), and need power (n P); and
     3) internal-external locus of control: individual-
     system blame and individual-collective action. The re-
     sults indicated support for the effects of self-esteem
     and internal-external control on life satisfaction
     among elderly Black adults. However, with the excep-
     tion of the findings for need power, the effects

(Peterson, John L.)

associated with need motivation were negligible. The
results were discussed in relation to several dynamic
theories of aging. The conclusion was offered that
future research should involve analysis of both
social-role and psychological effects of personality
on aging among Black adults.

Sears, June L. "Selected Environmental Factors Related
To Life Satisfaction of Black Senior Citizens." Unpublished Doctoral Dissertation, Michigan State University, 1975.

This study was designed to answer questions relative
to the degree of life satisfaction of low-income Black
elderly people and their relationship to the following selected environmental factors: nutrition, activities, interpersonal relationships, income and
health. The purposive, urban population sample selected consisted of 100 low-income Black men and
women 60 years of age or older. Each was living independently (not receiving convalescent or home care)
in either general or public housing or in a Senior
Citizens' Center within the city of Inkster, Michigan.
The feeling of life satisfaction among respondents
was notably high in terms of scores reported on the
life satisfaction index employed. Sixty percent
scored three-fourths (15 or more) of the items positively. These findings may be interpreted to mean
they were well satisfied with their lives. The study
provided some guidelines for identifying needs and
concerns of the elderly sample selected. It also
gave some insights as to their attitudes, perceptions,
and interests.

9. BLACK AGED AND HISTORICAL STUDIES

Pollard, Leslie J. "The Stephen Smith Home For The Aged:
A Gerontological History of a Pioneer Venture in Car-
ing For The Black Aged, 1864 to 1953." Unpublished
Doctoral Dissertation, Syracuse University, 1978.

The purpose of this dissertation is to provide historical perspectives of the Black aged. The emphasis on
the extended family has obscured a salient fact of the
Afro-American experience: that the Black community
provided a many-sided support of the elderly. A bal-
anced view of the care of elderly Blacks must include
mutual aid societies, benevolent associations and old
folks' homes. The dissertation is also designed to
fill a gap in gerontological literature by providing
a study of institutional care in an historical context. The involvement of Quakers in the Home sheds
greater light on an historic interracial contact.
Over 2,200 residents lived in the Home between 1865

(Pollard, Leslie J.)

and 1953. The great majority came from Philadelphia, having migrated there from such neighboring states as Virginia and Maryland. The Home was run under a dominant Quaker influence best described as paternalistic. Viewing the residents as children, the managers defined their needs and provided what they considered best for them. The writer argues that old age was viewed as a time of leisure, reflection, and preparation for death. Though some did not object to this concept of old age, others degenerated mentally in an atmosphere of resignation. Not a few clashed with administration, rebelling against enforced idleness and lack of stimulation. Since management denied work outside the Home, it emphasized entertainment, with an undue emphasis on religion. The author concludes that poverty and family breakdown were important factors that brought residents to live in the Home. Where relatives existed they were an important asset, providing personal care to the sick, engaging physicians, inquiring about proper treatment, and withdrawing the mentally ill.

Reilly, John T. "The First Shall Be Last: A Study of The Pattern of Confrontation Between Old and Young in The Afro-American Novel." Unpublished Doctoral Dissertation, Cornell University, 1977.

Most often the elder represents the protagonist's past, his heritage, and the ethos of his people, and the lessons he attempts to teach the protagonist are in sum the formidable and ubiquitous truths of Black life that he, himself, has learned from his experiences since slavery times. To survive, to define himself, to understand himself in relation to the world around him, to prosper, and/or to maintain his humanity, the protagonist is required to accept his elder's wisdom, or, in some way, to become reconciled with him. In a sense, his elder is the roots to which he, the young tree of Black life must be joined if he is to flourish. One of the significant facts disclosed by this dissertation is that while this pattern of confrontation somewhat varies from novel to novel, the concern for the Black heritage of struggle for freedom and advancement remains a constant.

Washington, Harold Thomas. "A Psycho-Historical Analysis of Elderly Afro-Americans: An Exploratory Study of Racial Pride." Unpublished Doctoral Dissertation, University of Massachusetts, 1976.

This is a study of racial pride across four historical periods based on retrospective interviews with elderly Afro-Americans. The four major Afro-American historical periods spanning from the 1890's to the present include: segregation, integration, Black power, and

(Washington, Harold Thomas)

Black nationalism. Three measures of racial identification were developed: racial pride scale, attitudes
toward Black leadership scale, and the leadership
awareness index. The general hypothesis reflecting
significant differences in leadership awareness across
the four historical periods was supported. The highest
assessment of leadership awareness was made during the
integration phase and the lowest assessment was made
during the Black power period. People from the higher
SES group were significantly more aware of Black leaders than people from the lower SES group in both the
integration period (t=3.06, p less than .01) and in
the Black power period (t=3.51, p less than .01). The
Southern sample was significantly more aware of Black
leadership than the Northern sample (t=4.13, p less
than .001).

10.   BLACK AGED IN SUBURBIA

Huling, William E. "Aging Blacks in Suburbia." Unpublished
    Doctoral Dissertation, University of Southern Cali-
    fornia, 1978.

The primary objective of this study is to provide qual-
itative information about the effects of culture on the
social organization of a Southern California suburban
Black community, known here as Pierce Park. Key social
systems of the mostly self-segregated enclave are examined for cultural patterns shared by a sample of aging, long-time residents who migrated to the community
in its formative years. A search is made for cultur-
ally-generated survival skills that have been used by
residents through their lifetime, and which can be expected to see them through old age. Comparisons between facets of Pierce Park's social organization and
those of other Black subcommunities identified in the
Cornell Studies of Intergroup Relations are made for
similarities and differences in cultural "universals"
found in them. Finally, cultural patterns are viewed
functionally; as they related to the maintenance of
survival skills and lifestyle in the community. A better understanding of the dynamics of an aging Black
community's social structure is provided from a Black
perspective. Migration was found to be a primary survival skill practiced by Blacks as a means of securing
a better quality of life. The church was found to be a
primary agent of migration, providing continuity between the old and new places of residence. Addition-
ally, the church becomes more active during periods of
crisis, and serves as a source of community cohesiveness and identity. It plays an important role in meeting the needs of the elderly. Cultural patterns are
strongly imbedded in the recreation and leisure systems of the community. Status is awarded to members

(Huling, William E.)

of the community based upon the quality of their participation in the recreation and leisure networks. Dormant survival skills are incorporated into leisure
activities, such as hunting, camping, and fishing. As
survival skills become dormant or unneeded, cultural
ties weaken between generations based upon a difference
in value systems. Interethnic relations vary with the
amount of perceived power; Blacks with little power mi-
grate away from interactions with Whites who have great
power, and remain in interactions with Mexican-Americans who have equal (or less) power. Perceptions of
old age are tied to health and activity rather than to
chronological age.

11.   COMPARATIVE AGED GROUPS

DeRidder, Joyce A. "Sex Related Roles, Attitudes, and Ori-
     entation of Negro, Anglo, and Mexican-American Women
     Over the Life Cycle." Unpublished Doctoral Disserta-
     tion, North Texas State University, 1976.

     The focus of this study is the relationship among (1)
     attitudes toward sex-based differentiation in adult
     leisure activities and socialization of boys and girls,
     (2) attitudes toward housekeeping, and (3) combinations
     of marital, maternal, employment, and head of household
     statuses among Negro, Anglo, and Mexican-American women
     in three categories and from two socio-economic levels.
     It is concluded that the lack of association between
     the two attitudinal variables and the role structure
     variable may be the result of the lack of refinement
     in the attitudinal and role combination measures, due
     to limitations of a secondary analysis of data. It is
     recommended that future studies direct attention to the
     differences created by ethnicity and various familial
     sex role constellations.

Gitelman, Paul. "Morale, Self-Concept and Social Integra-
     tion: A Comparative Study of Black and Jewish Aged,
     Urban Poor." Unpublished Doctoral Dissertation, Rut-
     gers University, 1976.

     In this study two distinct groups of aged, urban poor,
     Blacks and Jews, form the study population. The re-
     spondents reside in deteriorating urban areas, charac-
     terized by low income. Adjustment to old age was mea-
     sured by the major dependent variables, morale, self-
     concept and social integration, each subdivided into
     four dimensions. A questionnaire was constructed for
     the Jews through selection of items from Faulkner and
     Heisel's questionnaire with adjustments made for spe-
     cific group-related differences. Hypotheses were for-
     mulated regarding the relationship of designated ideal-
     types with dependent variables. From the findings it

(Gitelman, Paul)

is confirmed that religion, race and ethnicity have an impact on adjustment to old age. Current objective circumstances seem to be of secondary importance in regard to one's life satisfaction while levels of previous attainment provide important perspectives on life satisfaction. The writer states the position of the aged study group members as societal survivors is highlighted and the hypothesized strength of the married Jewish female, the stereotypical "Jewish Mother", is not confirmed. The limited utility of morale as a measure of actual need is indicated and the profound actual and potential impact of religion for the respondents is stressed.

12. COMPARATIVE BLACK AND WHITE AGED

Curran, Barbara W. "Getting By With a Little Help From My Friends: Informal Networks Among Older Black and White Urban Women Below The Poverty Line." Unpublished Doctoral Dissertation, University of Arizona, 1978.

The underlying assumption in this research was that ethnicity affects human behavior with respect to growing old. It was anticipated that differences resulting from ethnic factors could be observed in the ways respondents used formal and informal support systems. One hundred women, aged sixty or over, living in a Southwestern city, were interviewed. All had incomes below the poverty level and were living without marital partners. The sample was equally divided between Black and White women. Comparison between ethnic groups revealed substantially greater use of both formal and informal support systems by older Black women. Specifically, Black women made greater use of alternative medical systems, had larger networks of family and friends, participated at greater rates in institutional support systems, and rated themselves higher with respect to health and happiness than did White women. These differences were attributed to the closely cooperative life styles of Black women. These patterns of mutual support were thought to be a highly sophisticated cultural adaptation to historic and economic circumstances. While individual White women shared these cooperative values at times, as a group, patterns were at significant variance by ethnicity and White women appeared to exhibit independence, not interdependence. Other influential factors in this sample were discriminatory patterns of housing segregation for Black women and a rural southern background common to most Black respondents, but to only a few White women in the sample.

Davis, Dolores Jean. "Guide For Minority Aging Program at
     The Institute of Gerontology, University of Michigan:
     Student Perception Approach." Unpublished Doctoral
     Dissertation, University of Michigan, 1974.

     The purpose of this study was to develop a guide for a
     minority aging program at the Institute of Gerontol-
     ogy, University of Michigan (U-M). A twenty-five item
     questionnaire was constructed to assess U-M gerontol-
     ogy students' perceived needs, interests and atti-
     tudes related to (1) the need for additional minority
     aged curricula, (2) assessment of the present minority
     aged content in the U-M gerontology curriculum in
     meeting their educational and training needs, (3) per-
     ception of how these needs can be satisfied. The
     questionnaires were distributed in gerontology courses
     and/or mailed to all (120) gerontology students en-
     rolled during the 1974 spring term. The total re-
     sponse rate of 79, 15 Black respondents (100%) and 64
     White respondents (60%) was considered to be a normal
     distribution of U-M gerontology students for any
     given term. The guide for the minority aging program
     included the following recommendations: (1) A mini-
     mum of 20% of the gerontology curriculum should per-
     tain to the study of minority aging; (2) Minority
     aged content should be incorporated in all gerontol-
     ogy courses where appropriate and taught as special
     courses; (3) An Ethnicity and Aging course should be
     a required course for all gerontology majors; (4)
     Additional faculty with competencies in this area of
     specialization should be hired; (5) Recruit addi-
     tional minority students; (6) The three major compon-
     ents of the minority aging program should consist of
     research, training and service.

Gold, Joan Beth Klemptner. "A Study of Kinship Ties and
     the Institutionalized Aged: The Relationship Between
     Sources of Referral and Payment For Institutional
     Care of the Aged in Chicago, and Their Geographic Dis-
     tribution, Their Nearest Relatives, and Their Last
     Non-Institutional Address." Unpublished Master's
     Thesis, University of Illinois at Chicago Circle,
     1971.

     The title tells what this work is about. Various re-
     ferences are made to the Black aged throughout this
     work. The author points out that the racial composi-
     tion of the long-term care aged is overwhelmingly
     White (91 percent); non-Whites comprise less than 7
     percent. In 1960 8 percent of the aged population in
     metropolitan Chicago was non-White. Looking at the
     Black population only, the author found a larger pro-
     portion of males (36 percent) among this population
     than in the total institutionalized aged group. Six-
     ty-three percent of the Blacks have been referred by
     Public Aid while only 17 percent have been referred

(Gold, Joan Beth Klemptner)

by themselves or their families. This is due to a combination of factors, including the low socio-economic status of the Black population, contends Gold. The major source of payment for the Blacks makes it evident that social class is operating to some extent. Although only 63 percent had been initially referred by Public Aid, 75 percent are now having their care paid for by Public Aid; 10 percent are paid for privately and 15 percent by medical insurance and other sources. Since the Black population is different from the larger institutionalized group in several ways, special consideration was given to them in the analysis. The author states that for the Black population, referral source is not related to the distance variables, but major source of payment is. Blacks who pay privately live closer to nearest relatives but farther from their last non-institutional community than do Black Public Aid clients, concludes the author.

Ruberstein, Daniel I. "The Social Participation of The Black Elderly." Unpublished Doctoral Dissertation, Brandeis University, 1972.

This study was based on a subsample of 487 Black, 3419 White men and women 65 years of age and older from a national survey of elderly persons entitled Residential Physical Environment and Health of the Aged. The purpose of this study was to explore the social participation and well-being of the Black elderly (in comparison with the White elderly). Through the examination and analysis of data (obtained from personal interviews) the following objectives were addressed: (1) to describe the household situations and present an associational analysis of the participation of the respondents with their families and kin, friends and neighbors, and social organizations, and to measure the effect that this participation had on their morale or well-being; (2) to gather relevant information on the aged Black person; and (3) to relate the findings of this study to the provision of more effective social welfare services for the Black elderly through recommendations. The findings of this study suggested the following recommendations for programs for the elderly: (1) efforts should be made to raise income levels, and also Old Age assistance, as it is now practiced, should be replaced structurally by a less stigmatizing and more equitable and inclusive procedure of ensuring economic security; (2) the means of communication (telephone, transportation, etc.) for the Black elderly should be increased to expand opportunities for social interaction and social service; (3) group participation by the Black elderly should be encouraged and

(Ruberstein, Daniel I.)

discriminatory barriers against participation should
be eliminated; and (4) base line demographic data for
program planning and development should be developed
and further study and research on the Black elderly
sub-group in Social Gerontology should be encouraged.

Seelback, Wayne Clement. "Filial Responsibility and Morale
    Among Elderly Black and White Urbanites: A Normative
    and Behavioral Analysis." Unpublished Doctoral Dis-
    sertation, Pennsylvania State University, 1976.

This study is concerned with an examination of the
normative and behavioral dimensions of filial responsibility, and the bearing which these two dimensions
themselves and the congruence or incongruence between
them might have upon the morale of aged parents. The
sample consisted of 595 low-income, urban elderly,
seventy-five percent of whom were Black; their ages
ranged from sixty-five to ninety-nine. The data were
collected by teams of two or three interviewers who
were mostly indigenous to the neighborhoods in the
study. Data were analyzed by the Lazarsfeld Partial
Table Method, with square and gamma employed as measures of significance and strength of association,
respectively. Under both zero and first-order conditions, there were no significant racial differences in
a) type of expectation for filial responsibility, b)
levels of realized filial responsibility, or c) patterns of normative-behavioral congruence. However,
significant zero-order associations were found between type of expectations for filial responsibility
and age, marital status, income, health, and the extent to which a parent engaged in certain solitary
activities. Similarly, significant zero-order associations were also discovered between levels of realized filial responsibility and gender, marital status,
income, health and proximity of offspring. And also
at the zero-order level gender, marital status, income, health and solitary activity were significantly
associated with types of normative-behavioral congruence. A significant inverse zero-order association
was found between morale and types of filial responsibility expectations. This association was further
found to be conditional upon race, gender, age, marital and occupational statuses, solitary activity, religion, and proximity of children. Specifically, the
inverse association held only for Blacks, females, un-
married, low occupational status, low solitary activity, Protestants, and persons whose children lived
relatively near. Under zero and first-order control
conditions, morale was found independent of levels of
realized filial aid/support and types of normative behavioral congruence. The author concludes that the
fact that very few racial differences were found

(Seelback, Wayne Clement)

suggests that social class may be a more important
variable than color alone; given similar socioeconomic
conditions, Black and White family patterns in the
area of filial responsibility were relatively similar.

Stojanovic, Elisabeth J.   "Morale and Its Correlates Among
Aged Black and White Rural Women in Mississippi." Un-
published Doctoral Dissertation, Mississippi State
University, 1970.

It was the purpose of this study to assess the level
of morale of aged (60 and over) Black and White, low-
income, rural women and to determine the relationship
of their morale with activities and selected demographic, economic, social and attitudinal characteristics. The data were part of a larger nonage-strat-
ified sample of households in six low-income counties
in Mississippi, collected in 1961. The author concludes that Black women had relatively high morale.
They preferred outdoor activities, such as gardening
and fishing, as their pastimes. Better housing and
recreational facilities were among their expressed
needs. Self-reported place on the ladder was an important predictor of the self-image about statics
which in turn was significantly and positively correlated with morale. The White women did not appear
to possess the high morale displayed in the Blacks.
Their greatest concern was about their health. The
higher the activity score, the lower their morale.
They tended to engage in variety pastimes, especially
reading and television viewing. The latter was significantly and negatively correlated with morale and
was the most important predictor of morale.

Stone, Virginia. "Personal Adjustment in Aging in Relation
to Community Environment: A Study Of Persons Sixty
Years and Over in Carrboro and Chapel Hill, North Carolina." Unpublished Doctoral Dissertation, University
of North Carolina, 1959.

The author discusses the Black people of both Chapel
Hill and Carrboro that form a community between the
two boundaries of the towns, with the railroad track,
as usual, being one of the dividing lines. This
makes us have Community A, Chapel Hill White; Community B, the Black population; and Community C, the
Carrboro White. A census was conducted to determine
the number of persons who were 60 years and over. A
total of 910 people 60 years and over were located in
this area. The author found 552 in Community A, 206
in Community B, and 152 in Community C. In gathering
this information, she selected this on a demographic
basis, getting sex, age, and race. The oldsters of

(Stone, Virginia)

Community B were often the sons and daughters of
slaves. Most of these oldsters had substitute parents, and the father figure may have been completely
absent. It is this old Black who has built the family pattern that we are accustomed to. So, the old
Black still maintains more family control than either
of these White communities. In fact, very few of them
live alone--a small percentage of them are living
alone, 8.7 percent. Over one-fourth of them are living with relatives. One of the fascinating factors
about this is that the young Black moves in with the
old Black. The old Black owns the home, and since
the young move in with the old, the old Black maintains his role as head of the household. Hence, there
is not the same role change in this community as there
is in the other two communities. The old Black had
nothing to turn to outside of work but religion, and
religion offered him the outlet to release those
things that were pent up in him for so long. The
older Black of today is dissatisfied with the Black
church of today because "The church has gone fancy,"
and it doesn't provide him the opportunity for the
expression of emotionalism that the old church did.
One of the interesting things about the church pattern here is that the author found that the older
Black usually maintains his membership in the rural
church but comes under the watchcare of the town
church, so that he still has a tie with the church
that gives him a chance for expression. Throughout
the period of Reconstruction when the Black was having such a struggle, the one thing that he had to
hold to was God, so he has a tremendous belief in God
and the hereafter. In fact, they have been taught
all their lives that the one thing to live for is the
heavenly home, and this is what they are looking forward to. So when the Black gets old his morale goes
up instead of lowering as in most other people, because it won't be long before he can go to this
heavenly home, concludes the author.

Votan, Thomas E. "Death Anxiety in Black and White Elder-
     ly Subjects in Institutionalized and Non-Institution-
     alized Settings." Unpublished Doctoral Dissertation,
     Auburn University, 1974.

This study was designed to investigate the effects of
three variables on the level of death anxiety in an
aged population. The variables were: (1) Race
(Black vs. White), (2) Sex (male vs. female), and (3)
Institutionalization (institutionalized vs. non-institutionalized). A personality inventory was also utilized to examine the relationship between personality
factors and level of death anxiety. Eighty (80) elderly volunteers, equally divided with respect to the

(Votan, Thomas E.)

three variables, served as $\underline{S}$s. An effort was made to
control for age, mental and physical health, religion,
intelligence, length of institutionalization, and social class. Statistical analysis indicated that institutionalized $\underline{S}$s manifested significantly higher
death anxiety levels than non-institutionalized $\underline{S}$s
(p   .001), but the variables of race and sex had no
effect. Institutionalized $\underline{S}$s also showed significantly more "neurotic" symptomology than non-institutionalized $\underline{S}$s; correlation analysis revealed a significant positive correlation between level of death
anxiety and degree of neurotic preoccupation as measured by Mini-Mult scales: 1) (Hypochondriasis, r=
.28), 2) (Depression, r=.31) and 3) (Hysteria, r=
.29). Personality inventory differences were found
between Black and White $\underline{S}$s, but were interpreted with
caution due to recent evidence that postulates these
differences may well be due to subcultural differences rather than the idea that Blacks are more "pathological" than Whites.

5.

GOVERNMENT
PUBLICATIONS

1. BLACK AGED FEMALES

Jackson, Jacquelyne J. "Improving The Training Of Health
    Paraprofessionals." <u>Mental Health: Principles and
    Training Techniques in Nursing Home Care</u>. Margaret
    S. Crumbaugh, Editor. Rockville, Md.: National Insti-
    tute Of Mental Health, 1972, pp. 56-57.

This brief paper concentrates specifically upon one
group: nursing, housekeeping, and food service paraprofessionals employed or likely to be employed in the
South, the vast majority of whom are or are likely to
be Black females. Many of these Black females are
family heads or, if in husband-wife families, significant contributors to their total family income. Most
often, they labor diligently for wages at or below the
poverty level without even receiving minimally desirable fringe benefits, such as those of an established
period of two consecutive days away from and five days
at work during each week. Dr. Jackson feels strongly
that it is very important to initiate or upgrade training in mental health in these various curricula within
high schools, vocational schools, or other technical
training programs so that students would be certified
to work in the field following the completion of the
course or courses. Some attention should be given to
developing internship programs in conjunction with the
formal training on the high school level, underwritten
by such funds as those available from the Neighborhood
Youth Corps (NYC). Appropriate rewards--including pay
for internship in nursing homes under supervision--
should be included. Beyond that, there must be significant upgrading in wages and fringe benefits and fewer deadending jobs for such workers if there is to be
a real attempt to reduce heavy personnel turnover.
There may well be a need to consolidate smaller nursing homes, even if it means transferring residents or
potential residents to a larger complex since any home

(Jackson, Jacquelyne J.)

under 200 or so beds would be extremely unlikely to
provide an atmosphere especially conducive to training
and effective utilization of training as well as opportunity for upgrading personnel. Above all, attention must be given to defining precisely who is to be
trained by whom, for what, and when, where, and how,
argues Dr. Jackson. Currently, the author believes
that any training program designed for Black female
paraprofessionals should include training personnel
who are themselves Black.

2.   BLACK AGED AND THE FAMILY

Huling, William E. "Evolving Family Roles For The Black
    Elderly." Aging, September-October, 1978, pp. 21-27.

The author argues that historically, older Blacks have
provided a cohesiveness for the family by offering
both material and spiritual support to their children
and grandchildren. He further contends that the practice of treating the aged as assets rather than as
liabilities to the family has been demonstrated
through the years by Southern Blacks. The writer
states that the process of acculturation and assimila-
tion into the major social system is expected to di-
lute, if not destroy, both the traditional and cultural vestiges found in the Black family of past generations. Dr. Huling concludes that as more Blacks become urbanized, it appears that the persistence of
traditional roles for the Black aged is highly uncer-
tain.

3.   BLACK AGED AND HEALTH CONDITIONS

Jackson, Jacquelyne J. "Special Health Problems of Aged
    Blacks." Aging, September-October, 1978, pp. 15-20.

The author discusses primarily health perceptions, age
changes, prevalent diseases, functional health, and
the use of health resources as they relate to aged
Blacks. She argues that perhaps the most significant
issue is the conditions under which health resources
should be color-blind or color-specific for aged
Blacks. The writer states that health is a crucial
problem for most aged Blacks. Dr. Jackson concludes
that since the few Federal attempts to set forth research needs for aged Blacks in the past have generally ignored critical participants, including biomedi-
cal researchers, epidemiologists, health planners,
and health providers experienced in treating aged
Blacks.

Ostfeld, Adrain M.   "Nutrition and Aging--Discussant's Perspective." <u>Epidemiology of Aging</u>. Adrain M. Ostfeld and Don C. Gibson, Editors. Washington, D. C.: United States Government Printing Office, no date given. DHEW Publication No. (NIH) 75-711, pp. 215-222.

The writer points out that reliable data regarding diseases among aged Blacks are fragmented. Neither is much known about relationships between various conditions, such as obesity and strokes, nor between their morbidity. Recent mortality rates, based upon the underlying cause of death, show that diseases of the heart, malignant neoplasms, and cerebrovascular diseases account for about three-fourths of the deaths of all aged Blacks. The writer questions the traditional assumptions about undernutrition and overnutrition in older persons. Also some forms of heart or cerebrovascular diseases commonly thought to be affected substantially by obesity may not be so affected among the aged, concludes the author.

Shank, Robert E.   "Nutrition and Aging." <u>Epidemiology of Aging</u>. Adrian M. Ostfeld and Don C. Gibson, Editors. Washington, D. C.: United States Government Printing Office, no date given, DHEW Publication No. (NIH) 75-711, pp. 199-213.

The limited nutritional data available about aged Blacks suggest that their mean caloric intake is below standard, regardless of income level, as based upon body weight for age, sex, and height. Below standard, however, does not necessarily imply insufficiencies. The writer concludes that the diets of Blacks, 60 or more years of age, were characteristically low in iron, thiamine, and calcium, but they showed no serious deficiencies.

4.   BLACK AGED AND HOUSING

Johnson, Roosevelt.   "Barriers to Adequate Housing for Elderly Blacks." <u>Aging</u>, September-October, 1978, pp. 33-39.

Dr. Johnson concludes that if the Federal government is serious, prototype models can be developed and implemented to achieve the goals of adequate housing for elderly Blacks and to eradicate traditional barriers. Moreover, contends the author, the pervasiveness of racism and its negative effects will, by necessity, be lessened.

5. BLACK AGED AND INCOME

Lindsay, Inabel B., Editor, Consultant. U.S. Senate. Special Committee on Aging. The Multiple Hazards of Age
and Race: The Situation of Aged Blacks in the United
States. Report Number 92-450. Washington, D. C.:
U.S. Government Printing Office, September 1971.

The title tells what this work is about. The editor
states that statistics for 1971 on persons below the
low income level in 1971 indicate that almost twice as
many Blacks 65 years and over still fall below the low
income level (38.4 percent) as compared to the same
age group of Whites (19.9 percent). Dr. Lindsay contends that because of higher mortality rates for
Blacks and less longevity, a substantial number of
Black males in the age group 55 to 64, die before
reaching the age of eligibility for such social security benefits as they might be entitled to. She states
that a proposal for differentials in age eligibility
met considerable opposition, being called by some plea
for "preferential treatment." She also relates that
housing is another problem for the Black aged. According to the 1970 census, about 30 percent of the
housing units occupied by the elderly were judged substandard. For the Black elderly, the situation is
doubly distressing. In 1969, 63 percent of the Black
aged relocating in public housing were moving from substandard housing compared to only 30 percent of the
Whites who were relocating.

Orshansky, Mollie. "The Aged Negro and His Income." Social
Security Bulletin, Vol. 27, February 1964, pp. 3-13.

The writer contends that the income of the average
White worker is more sharply reduced in retirement
than the income of the Black worker, thus drawing the
two groups closer together in the common bond of strin-
gency. The author contends that for some time to come,
many Blacks reaching age 65 will continue to have limited resources and to be more dependent than White
persons on public aid.

Rubin, Leonard. "Economic Status of Black Persons: Findings From A Survey of Newly Entitled Beneficiaries."
Social Security Bulletin, Vol. 37, September, 1974,
pp. 16-35.

Information from the Social Security Administration's
Survey of Newly Entitled Beneficiaries was analyzed for
economic status differences between Blacks and Whites.
Black new beneficiaries were more likely than Whites to
become entitled to payable than to postponed benefits
and particularly to full rather than to reduced benefits. At whatever age they became entitled and what-

(Rubin, Leonard)

ever their payment status was, they were less likely
than Whites to have high PIA's (over $150) and retire-
ment pensions other than social security. Those whose
retirement income was limited primarily to social security benefits and whose PIA's were less than $150
subsisted at a level around the poverty line. Included in this low economic status were 88 percent of
the Black women, 62 percent of the Black men, 65 percent of the White women, and 32 percent of the White
men. The author concludes that earned income is especially important for those with inadequate retirement incomes, but low economic status was most often
associated with being constrained to stop work for
health or job-related reasons rather than with a positive desire to stop work. The relative disadvantage
of Blacks, and of women, was pervasive, holding for
every characteristic tabulated, states the writer.

Social Security Administration, Office of Research and Sta-
     tistics. "Current Medicare Report: Supplementary
     Medical Insurance--Utilization and Changes, 1972."
     Health Insurance Statistics, September 30, 1975.

     This article states that according to the HEW Medicare
     Survey Report for 1972, over half of the Blacks en-
     rolled in Supplementary Medical Insurance (SMI) either
     received no services or were not able to meet the de-
     ductible. In other words, the majority of elderly
     Blacks do not benefit from Medicare coverage because
     they cannot afford the payments, and over half of all
     poor elderly Blacks, whether living alone or in fami-
     lies, do not receive any Supplemental Security Income.

Thompson, Gayle B. "Black Social Security Benefits: Trends
     1960-1975." Social Security Bulletin, Vol. 38, April
     1975, pp. 30-40.

     Blacks and Whites are compared with respect to select-
     ed provisions of the OASDHI program--type of benefi-
     ciary, age of beneficiaries, size of benefits, and
     size of covered earnings--for the time period from
     1960-1973. There have been substantial increases in
     the number of Black beneficiaries since 1960, and in
     most beneficiary groups Blacks have increased propor-
     tionately more than Whites. The writer argues that
     Blacks are heavily represented among young benefici-
     aries but are underrepresented among aged beneficiar-
     ies. The average monthly benefit of Black benefici-
     aries was substantially below that of White benefici-
     aries in 1973, and the gap in benefit levels has nar-
     rowed only slightly since 1960. Several reasons for
     this discrepancy--the most important of which are dif-
     ferentials in the size of covered earnings and years

(Thompson, Gayle B.)

in covered employment--are discussed. He concludes
that discrepancies in benefit levels will persist for
some time, at least among men, because of continued
earnings within the younger generation.

6. BLACK AGED AND NURSING HOMES

"Home for Aged Colored Persons." Monthly Labor Review,
    August 1929, Vol. 29, pp. 284-288.

This is a study of Black Homes for the aged. A survey was made in 18 states and the District of Columbia. There were 33 homes that cared for 742 persons
at an annual cost of about $135,000. The largest num-
ber of persons, 185, were in Louisiana. This state
only spent $8,573. Pennsylvania, however, spent $42,
277 for 178 people. This article points out that generally speaking the physical conditions at the Black
homes did not equal those at the homes for Whites.
All of the Black homes, except one, had a Black matron
or superintendent.

Ingram, Donald K. "Profile of Chronic Illness in Nursing
    Homes, United States, August 1973-April, 1974." Vital
    and Health Statistics, Series 13, #29, DHEW Publica-
    tion (PHS) 78-1780. Hyattsville, Md.: National Cen-
    ter for Health Statistics, 1977.

The author points out that based upon a 1973-1974 survey, there were 49,300 Black residents of nursing
homes in the United States. This represents 4.6 percent of the total number of residents. Almost one-
fourth of them were under 65 years of age, although
only 11 percent of all residents were under that age.
Little more than over half of them were in the South.
The author believes that this figure may suggest that
aged Blacks may experience particular difficulties in
obtaining institutionalization within the South, or
that other factors, such as past memories of exclusion,
play a role.

U.S., Congress, Senate, Special Committee on Aging, Trends
    in Long Term Care, 92d Cong., 1st sess., 1972. Testi-
    mony by Hobart Jackson at public hearing on August 10,
    1971, pp. 2475, 2476.

Mr. Jackson points out that because of the universal
focus on providing alternatives to institutionalization for frail or otherwise dependent elderly, which
has been overlooked, is actually the reverse: "The
problem. . . is not one of how to keep the older Black
person out of a nursing home or similar institution,"
he said, "it is rather, how to get him or her in a
good one. . . ."

7. BLACK AGED POPULATION

Hill, Robert.   "A Demographic Profile of the Black Elderly."
    Aging, September-October, 1978, pp. 2-9.

The writer discusses population size, urbanization,
educational attainment, marital status, life expectancy, family composition, housing, amount of income,
poverty, sources of income, employment status, and
standard of living of the Black elderly. He argues
that the social and economic status of elderly Blacks
today are significantly better than they were a decade ago. Between 1970 and 1975, the life expectancy
of Blacks increased by almost three years and the gap
with Whites narrowed by at least one year. Thus,
there has been a sharp decline in the proportion of
elderly Blacks who are widowed. Dr. Hill concludes
that although elderly Blacks have made significant
strides, they still have a long way to go in achieving
an equitable and adequate quality of life.

United States Bureau of the Census. "Estimates of the
    Population of the U.S. by Age, Sex, and Race: 1970 to
    1977." Current Population Reports, Series P-25, No.
    721, 1978.

Since 1970, the Black aged population has been increasing more than twice as fast as the overall Black
population. While the total Black population increased by 11 percent, the number of Blacks 65 and
over increased by 25 percent--from 1.6 million to 1.9
million--raising the proportion of elderly persons in
the total Black population from 7 to 8 percent.

8. BLACK AGED AND POLITICS

Chunn, Jay. "The Black Aged and Social Policy." Aging,
    September-October, 1978, pp. 10-14.

The author declares that the social policy in the United States designed to serve the aged continues to
be fragmented and at times contradictory. He continues to state that a higher level of political consciousness must be developed for the elderly vote because politicians tend to respond to those constitu-
encies that vote together. The writer feels that the
presence of an adequate income level for aged Blacks
would help to alleviate many problems suffered by this
population. More adequate food could be purchased,
services would be more accessible through money for
transportation, more adequate housing could be maintained or secured and so on. He concludes that there
is a sense of urgency that should be recognized within the body politic of public policy as it determines
social policy outcomes. The quality of life of aged

(Chunn, Jay)

Blacks is, perhaps, declining, instead of improving.
The policy, programs, and services needed by the Black
aged and all elderly must ultimately be set forth and
must prevail in the public policy arena, contends the
author.

9.   MINORITY AGED

Koch, Hugo K. "National Ambulatory Medical Care Survey."
     Vital and Health Statistics, Series 13, #33, DHEW
     Publication (PHS) 78-1784. Hyattsville, Md.: Na-
     tional Center for Health Statistics, 1978.

The writer points out that in 1975, non-White aged
accounted for only 1.1 percent of all visits to of-
fice-based physicians in patient care. Of those who
visited, about 11 percent were new patients for the
specific physician, 18 percent were old patients with
new problems, and the remaining 71 percent were old
patients with old problems. The physicians felt that
about 31 percent of these patients had serious problems, about 36 percent, slightly serious problems, and
the problems of the remaining 33 percent were not serious, according to Hugo K. Koch.

U.S., Congress, Senate, Special Committee on Aging. A Pre-
     White House Conference on Aging. Summary of Develop-
     ments and Data. 92d Cong., 1st sess., 1971, Rpt.
     92-505.

This report stated that it is becoming increasingly
clear that the problem (of elderly Blacks in need) is
really one of multiple jeopardy, compounded by a
shortage of reliable statistical information on key
matters. In fact, this information gap has emerged
as a vital issue in all Committee on Aging research
related to minority groups, according to this report.

10.   COMPARATIVE BLACK AND WHITE AGED

Abbott, Julian. "Socioeconomic Characteristics of The El-
     derly: Some Black-White Differences." Social Secur-
     ity Bulletin, Vol. 40, July, 1977, pp. 16-42.

This article compares several characteristics of the
Black and White population aged 60 and older in March
1972. To distinguish race from economic-status effects the population is divided into quintiles of elderly units ranked by size of money income, and comparisons of selected demographic and economic characteristics are made within and across quintiles. Differences between social security beneficiaries and
nonbeneficiaries are also analyzed to ascertain the

(Abbott, Julian)

effects of social security benefits. The writer
states that the educational and occupational disadvantages of Blacks were evident even at the highest income level--a status more likely to be achieved by
married Black couples with both spouses working. The
author concludes that Black elderly units were less
likely than Whites to have social security benefits,
other government or private pensions, or income from
assets. They were generally more likely to have
earned income or to receive public assistance payments.

Mallan, Lucy B. "Women Born in the Early 1900's: Employ-
    ment, Earnings, and Benefit Levels." Social Security
    Bulletin, Vol. 37, March, 1974, pp. 3-16.

    In general, Black women earn much less than White
    women, and Black men earn much less than White men.
    Though both earnings and length of employment are
    higher for Black men than for Black women (as is true
    for White men and White women), the relative patterns
    are not the same. When the length of covered employ-
    ment since 1950 is examined, distributions for Black
    women and White women (and for Black men and White
    men) are the same, states Mallan. The writer argues
    when earnings are examined, however, a very different
    picture emerges. Median highest earnings for Black
    and White women and for Black men are, respectively,
    31 percent, 54 percent, and 63 percent of White men's.
    The author states earnings of Black men are closer to
    those of White women than to those of White men and
    about twice those of Black women. The author con-
    cludes these differences in earnings would have been
    even greater had the data included postponed as well
    as payable awards, since White men and women (with
    their higher earnings) postpone their awards more
    often than Black men and women postpone theirs.

Roberts, Jean. "Blood Pressure Levels of Persons 65-74
    Years, United States, 1971-1974." Vital and Health
    Statistics, Series 11, No. 203, DHEW Pub. No. (HRA)
    78-1648. Washington, D. C.: United States Govern-
    ment Printing Office, 1977.

    The author surmises that hypertension is more preval-
    ent among aged Blacks than Whites. She points out
    that between 1971-74 the prevalence rates per 100 for
    definite hypertension for persons 55-64 years of age
    were 54.5 for Black females, 49.9 for Black males,
    31.7 for White females, and 31.1 for White males; for
    persons 65-74 years of age, 58.8 for Black females,
    50.1 for Black males, 42.3 for White females, and
    35.3 for White males.

Thompson, Gayle B. "Black-White Differences in Private
    Pensions: Findings From the Retirement History Study."
    Social Security Bulletin, Vol. 42, February, 1979,
    pp. 15-40.

    This article compares older Black workers and older
    White workers on coverage under private pension plans,
    the receipt of pension benefits upon retirement, and
    the job characteristics associated with both coverage
    and receipt. Data are from the 1969 and 1975 inter-
    views of the Retirement History Study and describe
    pre-ERISA conditions among persons in their late fif-
    ties to mid-sixties. The author concludes that Black
    workers were much less likely than White workers to
    have been covered by a private pension on their long-
    est job. Moreover, among those who were covered, they
    were less likely to have received benefits. The ra-
    cial differences appear to result in part from sub-
    stantial differences on job characteristics, particu-
    larly industry, argues the writer.

United States Bureau of the Census. "Characteristics of
    Households Purchasing Food Stamps." Current Popula-
    tion Reports, Series P-23, No. 6, 1976.

    This article declares that during the peak of the 1975
    recession, only one-fifth of all elderly Black couples
    and one-fourth of all elderly Blacks living alone pur-
    chased food stamps, compared to 3 percent of all el-
    derly Whites living alone.

United States Public Health Service, National Center For
    Health Statistics. "Final Mortality Statistics,
    1976." Monthly Vital Statistics Report, Vol. 26, No.
    12, 1978, Supplement 2.

    This article states that, since 1970, Blacks have nar-
    rowed the life expectancy gap with Whites by at least
    one full year. In 1970, White men were expected to
    live to 68.0 years from birth, while Black men were
    expected to live only 61.3 years--a gap of 6.7 years.
    But by 1976, White men had a life expectancy of 69.7
    years, compared to a life expectancy at birth of 64.1
    years among Black men--a gap of 5.6 years.

White House Conference on Aging. "The Aging and Aged
    Blacks." Toward A National Policy on Aging, Vol. 2,
    Washington, D. C.: U.S. Government Printing Office,
    1971, pp. 177-196.

    The Black delegates at this conference were especially
    concerned with three major and related issues. One is
    the insufficient--and generally lack of attention
    given to minority groups, including Blacks, in the for-
    mation of issues presented at the conference. A

(White House Conference on Aging)

second issue was a general feeling of Black underrep-
resentation as Delegates and particularly so as linked
with other minority groups. Insufficient time to prepare and insufficient space to present their prelimi-
nary report constituted the third overriding issue.
It was also stated that the 1970 United States population contained 608,000 Black males 65 or more years
of age. Located in EVERY state, twice as many Black
aged as White dwelled in poverty; and one of every
two Black aged live in poverty. The delegates argue
that between 1959 and 1969, dollar income gaps between Black and White aged actually widened. Also
three of every four Black aged live in substandard
housing.

11. BLACK AGED AND THE NATIONAL
CENTER ON BLACK AGED

Faris, June B. (Editor). "Job Bank Lists Blacks In Field
of Aging." Aging, August, 1977, p. 24.

The National Center on Black Aged initiated a Job
Bank Service as a means of introducing Black professionals and paraprofessionals in the field of gerontology to employers seeking qualified personnel. The
Job Bank is a repository for information about positions currently available in the field of aging and
for the qualifications and backgrounds of persons
seeking employment. Applications will be screened and
those which match specified job descriptions will be
forwarded to employers. As a special feature, the
service includes assistance in the placement of older
persons seeking part-time, paid employment or volunteer positions in the field of aging. The Center has
as its primary concern the socio-economic needs and
welfare of aged Blacks. One of its major goals is
promoting the placement and advancement of Black professionals and paraprofessionals in the field of gerontology to meet these needs. NCBA is encouraging
employers and job seekers in aging and related areas
to utilize the service, which is free to members of
the organization. Prospective job candidates who are
not members of NCBA are charged $2.00 to cover postage
fees for one year from the date of registration.

6.

ARTICLES

1. BLACK AGED FEMALES

Clarke, John Henrik. "A Search For Identity." <u>Social Casework</u>, Vol. 51, No. 5, May, 1970, pp. 259-264.

In a moving personal account, the author tells of the forces and influences in his life that led him to develop creative and well-documented Black Studies. One of the forces that influenced him was his great grandmother, "Mom Mary," who had been a slave in Georgia and later in Alabama. Mom Mary was the historian of the author's family and told him stories about his family and how it had resisted slavery. Prof. Clarke concludes, "I think that my search for identity, my relationship to the world began when I listened to the stories of that old (Mom Mary) woman." He also recalls that she was a deeply religious woman and her concept of God was so pure and practical that she could see that resistance to slavery was a form of obedience to God. She thought that anyone who had enslaved any one of God's children had violated the very will of God.

Daly, Frederica Y. "To Be Black, Poor, Female and Old." <u>Freedomways</u>, Vol. 16, No. 4, Fourth Quarter, 1976, pp. 222-229.

The author argues that as Black women age, they who have experienced racism and sexism encounter in these most vulnerable, older years, the additional demeaning prejudice of ageism. For elderly Black women in this country, contends Day, too often men oversee their passage from "nigger" through "broad" to "old bag", a despicable history of deepening and widening unacceptability in direct ratio to the diminution of their strength as they grow old. The writer surmises that as if inadequate housing, poor health care and societal rejection were not enough, the elderly also

(Daly, Frederica Y.)

suffer from those who seemingly care yet refuse to
allow the elderly to share themselves and their accumulated life learning experiences with others. She
continues to assert that we need to bring pressure on
government to reorder our national spending priorities to include as major priorities programs that
will enhance the human quality of life for the elderly
poor. The author suggests that these programs should
include health reforms, expanded Medicare coverage,
manpower programs for older workers, health and nutrition education programs and for older workers, a
watchdog mechanism to prevent and punish swindling
and exploitation by those in the professions. She
concludes that individuals as advocates have the power
to do personal things that can help the elderly poor
such as asserting constant disapproval of ageism in
the neighborhood, on our jobs, in the media, wherever.
Further, advocates can help educate the elderly about
anti-discrimination laws and teach them how to identify illegalities and the agencies available to them
when they believe they are victims of ageism, sexism
and racism. Above all, the advocates must act as
publicists and facilitators, supporting the elderly's
rights to do for themselves, surmises the writer.

Gillespie, Bonnie. "Black Grandparents: Childhood Soci-
    alization." Journal of Afro-American Issues, Vol. 4,
    Nos. 3 & 4, Summer/Fall, 1976, pp. 432-444.

According to the author, as a result of this overall
study of Black grandparent and childhood socialization, the following conclusions have validity. 1.
Black grandparents traditionally and presently have
played a significant role in the socialization of
Black children and adolescents. 2. Telling stories,
family visits are several of the mechanisms through
which childhood socialization occurs via Black grandparents. 3. The Black extended family or multigen-
erational family exists today--although not in large
numbers, and grandparents play significant and important roles in such families. 4. The Black maternal
grandmother was indicated in this study as being the
main factor in Black childhood and adolescent socialization outside of the immediate nuclear family. 5.
The Black maternal grandmother in almost all instances
was viewed as a "second mother" and she treated her
grandchildren like they "were her own." 6. The male
respondents tended to have significantly greater affection and interaction with grandparents than the
female respondents. 7. The profile of selected grandparents by student respondents indicated a diversity
of education and occupation. Most tended to be female, Baptist, and Democrat. 8. The predominant relationship between Black children and grandparents

(Gillespie, Bonnie)

was one of "love," "affection," "compatibility," and
"dependability." 9. The Black church is an important link and socializing agent for Black grandparents
and grandchildren. 10. Today's modern American industrial society tends to have a detrimental effect on
Black grandparental relationships with grandchildren--
mainly due to mobility. 11. As a subset of the
Black elderly, on occasion, Black grandparents suffer
many of the inequities of this subpopulation via inadequate income: housing, and social/material environment. 12. Constructive work and programs for the
elderly have had a significant positive effect on the
elderly and their grandparent subset therein. 13.
The research of Black grandparental relationships,
effects on grandchildren, and the Black elderly is rewarding and intellectually stimulating to the Black
researcher, because it has great significance and implications for him/her, concludes Dr. Gillespie.

Himes, Joseph S. and Margaret L. Hamlett. "The Assessment
of Adjustment of Aged Negro Women in A Southern City."
Phylon, Vol. 23, Summer, 1962, pp. 139-147.

The article showed that although the 100 aged Black
women that were studied in Durham, North Carolina were
markedly in level of adjustment, they were concentrated at the upper end of the adjustment range. This
fact agrees with findings reported in other studies
of the aged, both Black and White, in both Southern
and Northern communities. Adjustment appeared to be
less adequate in the economic than in the social and
psychological areas, contend the authors. Differences
of level of adjustment were shown to be related significantly to variations of employment experience,
home ownership, education and health conditions. The
evidence from this and other studies suggests that
these variables comprise clusters of factors that are
significant in the experiences of aged persons. The
authors conclude that the women exhibited the greatest social adequacy in managing the household, social
participation, and personal decisions, and the least
in respect to exclusion from leadership roles. Psychological adjustment was best with respect to self
expression, reality definitions and self images, and
poorest with respect to role satisfaction. In the
economic sphere greatest adequacy of adjustment issued
from sufficiency of income and control of economic
activities, while most dissatisfaction came from inadequate income and lack of opportunity for training
and gainful employment, conclude the educators.

Jackson, Jacquelyne J. "Comparative Life Styles and Family and Friend Relationships Among Old Black Women."
Family Coordinator, Vol. 21, January, 1972, pp. 477-
485.

The total sample upon which this article was based
contained 74 women living with their spouse (hereafter married women) and 159 women without their
spouse (hereafter spouseless women), all of whom were
50 or more years of age. Data were collected in personal interviews in 1968-1969 from predominantly low-
income women representative of a Black, urban renewal
target area in Durham, North Carolina, and from a
nonrandom sample of middle-income women scattered
through or peripheral to that target area. The writer
declares that while the most important conclusion may
be the great similarity between these married and
spouseless women, the presence or absence of spouse
may be significantly related to such variables as number of close friends, sharing commercial recreation
with friends, dependence upon or participation with
children in emergencies of any sort and in shopping,
mutual assistance patterns between mothers and young-
est children, choices between spending more time with
friends or relatives, and specific preferences for
greater affinal or consanguinal contact.

_____. "Menopausal Attitudes and Behaviors Among
SENESCENT Black Women and Predictors of Changing At-
titudes and Activities Among Aged Blacks." Black
Aging, Vol. 1, August/October, 1976, pp. 8-29.

The author's major purpose in this article was to
share some hypotheses from an exploratory study of
a nonrandom sample of 51 postmenopausal Black women
about psychological and sociocultural events related
to the menopause. Emphasized most are relationships
between demographic variables and menopausal symptoms,
expected and occurred symptoms, and variables related
to attitudes about reproductive loss. Also considered
are symptomatic clustering and the women's use and
evaluation of medical treatment. Dr. Jackson points
out that a key explanatory concept for good social
and psychological adjustment in growing older for both
Black women and Black men, and for successful adjustment to menopause among Black women, may well be that
of social integration. The greater the integration
into social units meaningful to the individual and
the greater the individual's satisfaction with that
integration, the greater is her or his successful adjustment to aging. Growing older is generally more
successful when individuals share that continued aging with intimate others, and especially with satisfactory spouses.

Jackson, Jacquelyne, J. "The Plight of Older Black Women
in the United States." Black Scholar, Vol. 7, April,
1976, pp. 47-55.

This essay provided a cautious assessment of the
plights of economics, loneliness, mortality and iso-
lationism confronting aggregated older Black women as
they age in the United States. Although insufficient
data prevented any definitive assessment at this time,
minimal assessments relying both upon relevant demographic data and the writer's own value system were
possible and were so provided. Generally, the aggregated conditions of older Black women which were prevalent when they were younger continue into old age,
merely becoming more exacerbated. Perhaps the most
exacerbated plights related to those of insufficient
monies and insufficient men, states the writer. Dr.
Jackson surmises that there is a need to improve significantly not only the use of health care and delivery of preventive health care, but also to reexamine
seriously the extent to which the needs of older persons are met more effectively through organizations,
services, and other resources being based upon race,
sex, and age, et cetera, or upon more salient and
combinable characteristics. She concludes that this
is especially important for older Black women who have
for too long already been isolated from the central
core of longevity.

Johnson, Elizabeth F. "Look At It This Way: Some Aspects
of The Drug Mix-up Problem Among Blacks, Poor, Aged,
and Female Patients." Journal of The National Medical
Association, Vol. 70, No. 11, October, 1978, pp. 745-
747.

The author declares that elderly Blacks seldom have
sufficient funds to seek proper medical advice. They
frequently diagnose their own physical problems and
decide that they are minor. They are vulnerable to
slick Madison Avenue advertising that a pill or a drug
which can be purchased without a doctor's prescription
will give relief in a short time. This is especially
true of drugs advertised to give relief to the pains
of arthritis. And if one receives even the minimal
relief, the taking of the drug soon becomes habit-
forming, according to the author. The inability to
read labels with understanding continues to create
problems for persons with limited education, especially the elderly, concludes the writer.

Jones, Faustine C. "The Lofty Role of the Black Grandmother." Crisis, Vol. 80, January, 1973, pp. 19-21.

The author contends that the role of the grandmother
is one of love, strength, and stability for the Black

(Jones, Faustine C.)

family. She argues that no matter what social and
economic conditions the Black family has faced, the
Black grandmother has been a steady, supporting influence, as well as a connecting link between branches
of the extended family. Dr. Jones points out that
even during slavery the Black grandmother, during the
first five or six years of her grandchildren's lives,
sought to make them happy, comfortable, secure in her
love for them, and conscious of their worth in _her_
eyes. The writer surmises that there was no "generation gap" between the Black grandmother and her descendants after the era of slavery had ended. She concludes, it is clear that although the role of the
Black grandmother has changed and has been diminished,
she remains a source of love and strength as well as
a stabilizing factor for the Black family. The writer
continues to state that Black people, seeking to know
and appreciate their heritage, must understand the
role of the Black grandmother in the survival, growth,
and development of the Black family in America.

Penn, Nolan E. "Ethnicity and Aging in Elderly Black
    Women: Some Mental Characteristics," Health and
    The Black Aged. Wilbur H. Watson, et al., Editors,
    Washington, D. C.: National Center on Black Aged,
    1978, pp. 80-96.

    According to the author, aged Black and Indian women
    held more positive attitudes toward Children, "past"
    and "present," than did Caucasian women. In this
    sense, Black and Indian women did not seem to disen-
    gage; Black women held more positive attitudes toward
    parents in the "present" and "past" than did Caucasian
    and Indian women; and Caucasian women held more posi-
    tive attitudes toward work "past" and "present" than
    did Black and Indian women. In fact, Black women's
    attitudes toward Work were significantly more negative
    than those attitudes observed in the other two ethnic
    groups, concludes the writer.

Smith, Alicia D. "Life Satisfaction and Activity Prefer-
    ences of Black Female Participants in Senior Citizens'
    Centers: An Investigative Inquiry." Black Aging,
    Vol. 3, Nos. 1 and 2, October and December, 1977,
    pp. 8-13.

    This study was conceived of as an investigative in-
    quiry into the life satisfaction and learning prefer-
    ences of Black older adults. The purpose was to ob-
    serve and report on behavioral issues which effect
    aging adjustment. Measurements were made of individ-
    ual life satisfaction and additional data was col-
    lected on personal motivation for utilizing the cen-

(Smith, Alicia D.)

ter, responses to a list of activities, and on the
perceptions of both participants and administrators
with regard to the needs of the elderly. Fifty participants and four administrators, at four centers,
were identified. The results of this inquiry indicate
that three variables: age, health and length of residency are significant correlates of life satisfaction
and that length of residency is the single best predictor of satisfaction. The indications are also that
members prefer health and personal oriented activities. It is concluded that cultural experiences and
values play a significant role in defining individual
needs, and that for this population, aging adjustment
means engaging in and enlarging upon social interactions and experiences rather than disengaging, concludes the author.

2. BLACK AGED AND FAMILIES

Jackson, Jacquelyne J. "Family Organization and Ideology."
Comparative Studies of Blacks and Whites in The United
States. Kent S. Miller and Ralph M. Dreger, Editors.
New York: Seminar Press, 1973, pp. 405-445.

One section is devoted to the "Aged Roles and Statuses." Dr. Jackson argues that it appears that effective kinship networks characterize the family lives of
both aged Blacks and aged Whites, that parental and
child sex preferences persist into aged parent-adult
child relationships, and that there are presently no
significant differences by sex between the two racial
groups as measured by their marital statuses and by
the proportions who live alone and do not live alone.

_____. "Marital Life Among Aging Blacks." Family
Coordinator, Vol. 21, January, 1972, pp. 21-27.

The writer states that while this article has focused
specifically upon selected marital patterns among
married aging Blacks, much more attention must also be
given to those supportive familial patterns available
for aged Black males and females without spouses. At
present, it appears that such individuals still depend, as they have in the past, upon their own families as the first line of resource or assistance.
When they have children, they turn toward them, and,
most often, their children respond. In the absence
of children, they direct their needs toward other relatives, and those relatives respond as well. It thus
appears that family functioning among Blacks is still
highly supportive, to the extent possible, for aged
family members. Dr. Jackson asserts ineffective family functioning which may occur can best be attributed

(Jackson, Jacquelyne J.)

to the lack of strongly societal factors. The author
concludes a guaranteed annual income providing at
least a moderate living for aging and aged Blacks,
and other non-Blacks in need, may be a step in the
right direction. It can help strengthen family functioning for aged Blacks, declares Dr. Jackson.

_____. "Kinship Relations Among Older Negro Ameri-
cans." Journal of Social and Behavioral Sciences,
Vol. 16, 1970, pp. 5-17.

This article has three major purposes. The first is
the proffering of some cautious and categorical generalizations about older Blacks. The second is that
of providing some findings about specific kinship
relations among a specific sample of older Blacks.
The third is that of commenting upon some of the implications of these generalizations and findings as
they may relate to the concept of racial subculture
in kinship relations among older Americans. Dr. Jackson argues that essentially, kinship of relations
among older Black Americans displayed no gross struc-
tural and functional differences from those of other,
older Americans. She concludes that despite the wide
communication given to the "increasing polarization
of Black and White," the increasing separation between Black America and White America, it appears to
her that the concept of racial subculture, when employed in descriptions and analyses of kinship relations of older persons in the United States, is of
relatively little conceptual value.

3. BLACK AGED AND CHILDREN

Jackson, Jacquelyne J. "Sex and Social Class Variations
in Black Aged-Parent-Adult Child Relationships."
Aging and Human Development, Vol. 2, August, 1971,
pp. 96-107.

This article deals with a pilot investigation involving thirty-two aged Black parents and their eighty-
three adult children. It revealed that significant
sex and social class differences were apparent with
respect to patterns of instrumental aid to and from
these parents and their children, as well as their
affectional relationship. She concludes that most of
the Black aged surveyed did not consider themselves
nor their children as mutual sources of moral support,
with the major exceptions of manual fathers and their
daughters and nonmanual fathers and their children;
but nonmanual parents were more likely to perceive
themselves in this regard than were manual parents,
as was true of fathers more often than of mothers.

Jackson, Jacquelyne, J. "Negro Aged Parents and Adult
    Children: Their Affective Relationship." Varia,
    Spring, 1976, pp. 1-14.

    Essentially, the focus of this article was that of
    sharing certain findings, and hypotheses derived
    therefrom, obtained in a pilot investigation of aged
    Black parents' perceptions of their affective involve-
    ment with their adult children, and of some of the
    factors which affect such involvement. Dr. Jackson
    surmises that theoretically, the data tended to sug-
    gest that common cultural interests and affection may
    be sufficiently binding to provide continuity and
    substance to those parent and child nuclear families
    maintaining economic self-sufficiency, but that, in
    the absence of such self-sufficiency, affection and
    common cultural interests were not sufficiently bind-
    ing to provide such continuity and substance. Thus,
    it appears that economic self-sufficiency is a varia-
    ble with significant implications for aged parent-
    adult child emotional or affective relationships,
    states Dr. Jackson. The author declares that the data
    tends to suggest that more attention ought to be
    placed upon the social relationships or role inter-
    actions, as well as role structures, and the meanings
    which such role interactions have for the partici-
    pants as indicated by the participants, as well as
    their quantity, in studying not only Black aged par-
    ents and their children, but also in studying gener-
    ally the Black family. The writer concludes that as
    might have been expected on the basis of other liter-
    ature not cited herein, the pilot investigation indi-
    cates that, in all probability, most aged Black par-
    ents prefer to live independently of, but in close
    contact with, their children; that, in those situa-
    tions defined as "crises," most such parents assist
    or are assisted by their children; that most such
    parents tend to prefer a daughter, as opposed to a
    son; and that their affectional involvement with or
    their affects toward their children are influenced by
    a number of variables, not the least of which are the
    sex and socioeconomic status of the parent and the
    child, the early parent-child relationships, and de-
    gree of dominance or authority by either parent or
    child within their present relationships, concludes
    Dr. Jackson.

Pihbald, C. T. and Robert W. Habenstein. "Social Factors
    in Grandparent Orientation of High School Youth,"
    Older People and Their Social World, Arnold M. Rose
    and Warren A. Peterson, Editors. Philadelphia: F. A.
    Davis Co., 1965, pp. 163-180.

    This essay is based on the assumption that kinship
    ties in the contemporary family are directly related
    to the degree of knowledge held by grandchildren of

(Pihbald, C. T. and Robert W. Habenstein)

their grandparents. The authors compared White and
Black high school youths. They concluded that more
than twice as many White as compared with Black students were able to report the occupations of both
grandfathers. The writer also states that only one-
fifth of the White students as compared with half the
Blacks reported the occupation of neither grandfather.

4.   BLACK AGED AND HEALTH CONDITIONS

Calloway, Nathaniel O.   "Medical Aspects Of The Aging Amer-
ican Black." Proceedings of Black Aged in The Future,
Jacquelyne J. Jackson, Editor. Durham, N. C.: Center
For The Study of Aging and Human Development, Duke
University, 1973, pp. 50-56.

The writer focused on two themes in this paper. First,
he gives a brief description of the overall health of
aged Blacks and some needed research. Second, he compared selected non-White with White life expectancies,
and mortality rates and causes. Dr. Galloway argues
that currently (1973) old Blacks represent a biologi-
cally superior population in comparison with younger
Blacks and old Whites, primarily because they represent SURVIVORS of a cohort group detrimentally oppressed by various hazards who were able to adjust and
adapt in various ways to their environments. The author concludes that better health statues in the
younger years will contribute to longer Black life-
expectancies and, of course, larger populations of
aged Blacks, but will not, at present, contribute to
longer life spans.

Greene, D. Richard.   "Health Indicators and Life Expectan-
cy of the Black Aged: Policy Implications,"
Health and The Black Aged, Wilbur H. Watson, et al.
Editors. Washington, D. C.: National Center on
Black Aged, 1978, pp. 31-45.

This article focused on vital statistics, including
mortality data, as indicators of the differential
health statuses of older persons. As conditional factors, the author included sex and residence according
to census tract. A major difference between this
study and others was its focus on a local metropolitan community. This approach was intended to reduce
some of the data ambiguities inherent in national
studies. The writer used vital statistics from 1969-
70 along with 1970 census data for the City of Seattle,
Washington. Ten thousand records of vital statistics
were available for analysis. The aim of the study was
to develop a framework for policy recommendations and
appropriate interventions for the reduction of race-

(Greene, D. Richard)

related mortality differentials. Greene contends that
policy should reflect obvious and more subtle factors
which relate to race-related differences in longevity
and their implications. The writer found that the
older patients had a larger proportion of conditions
that were due to degenerative vascular diseases and
the younger ones had more diagnoses related to trauma.
The author was able to demonstrate that with advancing age there was decreasing functionability as reflected in the statistically significant lower frequency with which older persons left their homes.
This latter finding suggested that the older group may
have had other sub-clinical chronic conditions that
were related to the major rehabilitation diagnoses and
that were expressed in lower levels of functioning.

Hawkins, Reginald. "Dental Health of Aged Blacks." Pro-
    ceedings of Black Aged in The Future . Jacquelyne J.
    Jackson, Editor. Durham, N. C.: Center for The Study
    of Aging and Human Development, Duke University, 1973,
    pp. 57-77.

The writer surmises that there is an alarming number
of older Blacks needing early dental care. Among
those 55-64 years of age, 78.5 percent of Black males
and 79.2 percent of Black females needed such care.
He concluded that dental health care is generally poor
for most Blacks, and it tends to become increasingly
poor with age. Dr. Hawkins also points out that those
interested in curriculum building for the aged must
also be interested in increasing the number of Black
dentists available to treat aged Blacks.

Henry, Melvin. "Perceived Health Status of the Black El-
    derly in an Urban Area: Findings of a Survey Research
    Project." Health and The Black Aged. Wilbur H. Watson,
    et al, Editors. Washington, D. C.: National Center
    on Black Aged, 1978, pp. 72-79.

The author's findings indicated that elderly Blacks in
the Los Angeles area did not fit the commonly held
stereotype of the Black elderly as feeble, dependent,
decrepit, emaciated, generally in poor health and
people who are worse off than any other group in the
society. Further, the elderly in the author's sample
seemed to have very few problems in gaining access to
available health care services; they were infrequently
represented on the rolls of public welfare and lists
of persons receiving Supplemental Security Income.
The majority of the Blacks in this sample rated their
health as very good, good, or fair and believed that
their health was at a level equal to or better than
that of other people their own age. Functionally,
these elderly Blacks were able to take care of routine

(Henry, Melvin)

activities of daily living and experienced little or
no problems in getting good medical treatment. The
costs for medical care were covered by government programs or private insurance. The majority of the respondents attributed responsibility for securing
health care for the elderly to the federal level of
government. In general, this sample of Black elderly
reported few problems relative to health care. The
major areas of concern were restricted employment and
mobility. In particular, there were difficulties in
holding a regular job and walking up three flights of
stairs. Some also reported insurance problems involving difficult instructions and explanation of benefits, long delays in receiving reimbursement for
medical expenses and transportation problems concludes the author.

Jackson, Jacquelyne, J. "Action and Non-Action." Action
For Aged Blacks: When? A Conference of The National
Caucus on The Black Aged. Washington, D.C.: National
Caucus on The Black Aged, 1973, pp. 12-17.

The writer discusses the history of the National Caucus on The Black Aged beginning with its origins in
1971. She states that some of the programs that effect Black people and specifically older Blacks are
only receiving "piecemeal" money for their support.
Since various Black groups are competing for the
"same monies" to keep their programs going, in terms
of action or nonaction, they get caught in the game
of divide and conquer, argues Dr. Jackson. She also
points out that the absolute gap between old Blacks
and old Whites has not only continued to increase
over the past several decades but is continuing to increase.

Kovi, J. et al. "Gastric Cancer in American Negroes."
Cancer, Vol. 34, No. 1, July, 1974, pp. 765-770.

There were 110 males and 40 females in this study, a
male to female ratio of 2.75:1. A number of American series of stomach cancer have reported male pre-
dominance in sex ratios ranging from 2.6:1 to 2.0:1.
The patients' ages ranged from 25 to 87 years. The
mean age for males was 62.3 years and for females was
64 years. Corresponding figures for American Caucas-
ians were 65.0 years for males and 62.1 years for females. This study was done at Howard University Hospital.

Lewis, Edward A. "High Blood Pressure, Other Risk Factors
    and Longevity: The Insurance Viewpoint." American
    Journal of Medicine, Vol. 55, September, 1973, pp.
    281-294.

The author points out that in the United States, the
proportion of Black men aged 45 to 65 with distinctly
elevated systolic or diastolic blood pressures appears to be about double that of White men. In Black
women aged 45 to 54, the proportion with such elevated
blood pressures is about two and a half times that
among White women; however, among Black women aged 55
to 64 the proportion with distinctly elevated pressures
is only about a third higher than among White women.
This is because the proportion of hypertensive Black
women is rather high at ages under 45 and does not increase with advancing age as sharply as in White women among whom the prevalence of elevated blood pressures at ages under 45 is relatively low. The higher
blood pressures of Blacks do appear to be related to
their generally lower socioeconomic status. This was
brought out in a study of the race differentials in
mortality attributed to hypertension in which the
blood pressures of Whites and non-Whites in various
occupations and at various income levels were compared;
the mortality from hypertensive disease was much higher in non-Whites regardless of occupation or socioeconomic class. A number of investigations disclose
a wide variation in blood pressure levels among different racial and ethnic groups. It has been suggested that the higher blood pressures noted among Blacks
in the United States may reflect a genetic factor.
This conclusion is based partly on observations that
hypertension is quite common in West African tribes,
whereas average blood pressures in several East African tribes resemble more nearly those of Whites in the
United States, surmises the writer. Average blood
pressures distinctly higher than those among Blacks in
the United States have been recorded in young Poly-
nesians and Melanesians, concludes the author.

Lewis, Irene. "The Study of Hypertension Compliance in a
    Group of Elderly Third World Patients." Health and
    The Black Aged. Wilbur H. Watson, et al., Editors.
    Washington, D. C.: National Center On Black Aged,
    1978, pp. 4-17.

The article focuses on identifying factors that could
be relied upon to indicate a patient's potential for
high compliance with a treatment plan for hypertension.
The author attempted to determine whether any such
factors could be manipulated by the provider to increase the likelihood of compliance. Each patient's
compliance with a treatment plan was assessed infor-
mally. The degrees of compliance were loosely put as

(Lewis, Irene)

"low," "medium," and "high." Out of nine cases, one person was judged low, three as medium, and five (5) as high compliers. Recent audits of patient records at the clinic where the author conducted this study showed that her findings were generally representative of compliance behavior.

McDowell, Arthur. "Health Data On Aging Persons." Proceedings of The Research Conference on Minority Group Aged in the South. Jacquelyne J. Jackson, Editor. Durham, N. C.: Center for the Study of Aging and Human Development, Duke University Medical Center, 1972, pp. 117-124.

The author states that the prevalence of heart disease is higher for Blacks than Whites. About 16 percent of the adult White male population has heart disease of all types, as compared with about 36 percent of their Black counterparts. A stronger differential exists comparing the older adult population by race. Hypertension shows a White male prevalence rate of about 18 percent and a Black male rate of about 37 percent. Corresponding data are 21 percent for White and 40 percent for Black females. Over and over again you see this difference. Really significant is the concealed classification such as income. There you see much of the apparent racist difference as an income difference. Much the same is true of such other measures as limitation of activity. About two-fifths of those 65+ years of age suffer a limitation in their ability to do their regular work or housework due to some chronic condition, with a clear racial differentiation unfavorable to Blacks, states the author. While there is not such a clear differential in the 45-64 year-old group or at least not quite a big rate when the age group under consideration is broadened you are still looking at limitation of activity related to income. There is a very clear relationship. More chronic conditions cause greater disability among the poor, concludes the author.

Newman, Gustave, et al. "Alterations in Neurologic Status With Age." Journal of the American Geriatrics Society, Vol. 8, No. 12, December, 1960, pp. 915-917.

The 200 persons studied were volunteers who lived in the community in and around Durham, North Carolina. Their ages ranged from 60 to 93 years (average 70 years). Males and females of both the White and Black races were included. The neurologic examination was conducted using only the more common standard tools, such as a reflex hammer, a tuning fork, a straight pin and some cotton. The findings were recorded in the usual clinical manner, that is, as indicating normal,

(Newman, Gustave, et al.)

moderately impaired function, or severely impaired
function. Of 27 items from the neurologic examination, the 9 which presented the greatest number of
deviations from normal were selected for closer scru-
tiny. These variables were gait, reflex activity,
movements associated with gait, involuntary movements
(tremor), vibratory sensibility (128 tuning fork),
two-point discrimination, touch, pain and olfaction.
The writers argue that variables such as palsies of
the cranial nerves were of such infrequent occurrence
as to be of no value in a statistical study. The
foregoing 9 neurologic variables were cross-indexed
against the 4 basic demographic variables of sex,
race, age and socioeconomic status, and tested for
significance of variability by the chi square test.
It was pointed out that alterations of reflex activity
were much more highly correlated with race, the White
subjects tending to be hyper-reflexive, whereas the
Blacks were hypo-reflexive. This racial difference
was statistically much more significant than the sex
difference, and had a P value of .001; that is, the
probability was 1 in 1,000 that it was due to chance,
conclude the authors.

Nichols, Gloria J. "Drugs and Nutrition." Journal of the
     National Medical Association, Vol. 70, No. 10, Octo-
     ber, 1978, pp. 737-738.

According to the writer, in our society, the elderly
are the principal drug users. Patients over 65 make
up somewhat less than 11 percent of the population,
but they spend more than 25 percent of all monies ex-
pended for drugs. They may take prescription medications for the treatment of one or more diseases or
they may self-medicate for symptoms associated with
old age. The elderly spend a great deal of time
watching television, where they are bombarded by com-
mercials with claims that a particular pill can re-
lieve an aching back, indigestion, swollen legs, or
some other distressing health problem. They will often go to the corner drugstore for medications hoping
to get instant relief. Excessive use of laxatives by
older people may be due to the widespread, but erron-
eous, belief that one must have daily bowel movements
and that simple constipation resulting from improper
diet must be controlled with laxatives, contends the
author. The elderly constitute a subgroup in which
nutritional depletion or malnutrition is prevalent.
Many factors predispose them to nutritional deficiencies, including lack of knowledge about drugs they
are taking, foods that should be avoided or included
in their diet, social isolation, physical disability,
mental disturbance, and poverty. As secondary factors,

(Nichols, Gloria J.)

dulled taste buds, false teeth, and irregular cooking
habits contribute to inadequate diets. A drug can be
potentiated by an empty stomach or an undernourished
body. Aging is associated with many chronic diseases
that can reduce appetite, cause malabsorption, and decrease nutrient utilization. Such diseases include
congestive heart failure, diabetes, and cancer. Because of the pathophysiological changes produced by
aging, elderly patients tend to absorb drugs at a
slower rate, distribute them differently, and eliminate them less efficiently than middle-aged patients,
concluded the author.

Nowlin, John B. "Successful Aging: Health and Social Factors In An Inter-Racial Population." Black Aging,
Vol. 2, Nos. 4-6, April, June and August, 1977, pp.
10-16.

This article proposes a tentative definition of "successful aging" and examines data collected from an
older population in the context of this definition.
Any specific definition of "successful aging" will
necessarily be, at least in part, arbitrary, states
the author. Two criteria, both with primie facie validity, would be chronologic age itself and health status. With respect to chronologic age, the older person, by virtue of remaining alive and accruing years,
reflects some degree of success in dealing with vicissitudes of aging. The particular age at which an individual can be considered "successful" in coping with
these "vicissitudes" is moot. Yet another geronto-
logic "talking point," at present equally informal as
that of "successful aging," is consideration of later
life in terms of "younger old-age" and "older old-
age"; the age of 75 has been suggested as the dividing
point between these two age groups, according to Nowlin. Attainment of age 75 then could serve as a reasonable age criterion for definition of "successful
aging." Other than chronologic age, it is difficult to
conceive of a factor more fundamental to any notion of
"successful aging" than health status. The pervasive
role of health in all aspects of coping for any age
group needs little emphasis. Since senescence itself
often is associated with loss of physiologic resources, health status seems an obvious second criterion
for "successful aging," concludes the author.

Primm, Beny J. "Poverty, Folk Remedies and Drug Misuse
Among the Black Elderly." Health and The Black Aged.
Wilbur H. Watson, et al., Editors. Washington, D. C.:
National Center on Black Aged, 1978, pp. 63-70.

The writer points out that pharmacists must be alerted
to the problems of possible over-medication resulting

(Primm, Beny J.)

from prescribed and over-the-counter drugs. Physicians must learn to care for the elderly, not just cure them: (1) They must take time to talk to their patients; (2) They must explain the condition for which a drug is prescribed; and (3) They must look for inexpensive, generic (not brand name) drugs to prescribe. In sum, they must teach prevention. State and national legislators must rectify some basic problems in this area by law. For example, every drug sold in America for senior citizens should be required to state, in large type, exactly what the consumer should know: How many to take, what not to take it with, et cetera. A comprehensive national health plan would also help. Health care must be a right, not a privilege, concludes the author.

"Sam Johnson Is Still Horsing Around at 99," _Jet_, November 22, 1973, pp. 62-63.

Article concerns a 99 year old ex-slave who worked as a stablehand, exercise boy, a one-race jockey, trainer and groomer for 81 years. He credits "soul food" for much of his good health. "Soul food ain't nothing new. It's older than me," reminded Johnson. At 99 years old he still walked at least one mile a day-- in morning and evening installments from his home in Elmont, Long Island, N. Y., to Belmont Park race track and back.

Shafer, Stephen Q. "Brain Infarction Risk Factors In Black New York City Stroke Patients." _Journal of Chronic Diseases_, Vol. 27, 1974, pp. 127-133.

The author points out that of 527 consecutive stroke patients at Harlem Hospital, 22 percent had had a previous stroke: 57 percent had hypertension: 28 percent had diabetes mellitus: 24 percent had advanced heart disease: 18 percent had none of these conditions identified. These proportions match those from White series, except for the low prevalence of heart disease, which was recorded only in clinically symptomatic stages. When the series was divided in half by age, diabetes, heart disease and previous stroke were each more common in patients 65 and older. Hypertension was significantly (p is less than 0.02) less frequent. The Health Examination Survey estimated that 52 percent of Blacks age 65-74 and 60 percent of those aged 75-79 are hypertensive. In Harlem stroke patients, by contrast, the prevalence of hypertension at ages 65-74 was 48 percent. It fell to 37 percent for ages 75 and over. In more aged patients, hypertension seemed to be less common than estimates.

Shafer, Stephen Q. et al. "The Contribution of Nonaneurys-
    mal Intracranial Hemorrhage to Stroke Mortality in New
    York City Blacks." Strokes, Vol. 4, November/Decem-
    ber, 1973, pp. 928-932.

The authors surmise that of 527 unselected stroke patients (98% Black) in a New York City hospital, 80
(17%) had nonaneurysmal intracranial hemorrhages, with
a fatality rate of 85%. Of 216 inhospital deaths 37%
were due to such hemorrhages. In patients aged 65 and
less, 52% of 90 fatal events were hemorrhagic. Only
in patients below age 46, however, did cerebral hemorrhage account for more deaths than infarction. The
incidence of hemorrhage and the proportion of inhospital deaths from it were higher than in three White
American and lower than in one Black African series.
The differences were not major, and could be explained
by varying definitions and hospital use. The mean age
of patients with fatal hemorrhage was 61 years. When
the inhospital mortality is extrapolated into annual
mortality estimates, the following conclusions according to the authors may be drawn about spontaneous nonaneurysmal intracranial hemorrhage in New York City
Blacks: (1) above age 45, it does not account for more
deaths than infarction, (2) it is not much more common or lethal in Blacks than in Whites, and (3) it
does not occur more predominantly at earlier ages in
Blacks than in Whites.

Staggers, Frank. "Carcinoma of the Prostrate Gland in
    California: A Candid Look at Survival Trends in Re-
    gards to Stage, Race and Social Class." Health and
    The Black Aged. Wilbur H. Watson et al., Editors.
    Washington, D. C.: National Center on Black Aged,
    1978, pp. 18-30.

Cancer of the prostate is the most frequent category
of all cancers occurring in Black males after the age
of 65, states the author. The presence of the disease can be detected by rectal examination. As indicated by the California Tumor Registry for Alameda
County between 1942 and 1969, White males with cancer
of the prostate seemed to have had a higher survival
rate than Black males, according to Staggers. However, when type of treatment setting was controlled,
White males treated in county hospitals had a lower
survival rate than all other groups, including Black
males. The author concludes that while it was clear
that there were race-related differences between
Black and White males in the rate of cancer of the
prostate, there were also differential treatment effects that may have reflected class and technological
differences between intervention systems when patients
were admitted to private versus county (public) hospitals.

Thompson, Larry W. et al. "Relation of Serum Cholesterol
    to Age, Sex, and Race in an Elderly Community Group."
    Journal of Gerontology, Vol. 20, 1965, pp. 160-164.

Total serum cholesterol determinations were made on
198 elderly persons (60-93 years) living in or around
Durham, N. C., as part of a comprehensive study of human aging. Repeat determinations were obtained on 74
of these people after a three-year interval. White
and Black community volunteers of both sexes and a
wide range of socio-economic levels were included.
No over-all age effect was observed. Females in their
seventh and eighth decades had significantly higher
serum cholesterols than males, but sex differences
were less pronounced in the oldest group (80-93
years). The data suggest that females reach a peak
value in their 60's followed by a gradual decline,
while males above 60 undergo little change with time,
state the authors. A sex by race interaction was also apparent, with the Black males having significantly higher levels than the White males; the difference
between White and Black female groups was minimal according to the writers. A comparison of Ss with and
without clinical evidence of cardiovascular disease
revealed no differences, which suggests that cholesterol level may play a less significant role in the
development of pathological processes in senescence
than in middle age.

Weaver, Jerry L. "Personal Health Care: A Major Concern
    For Minority Aged." Comprehensive Service Delivery
    System For The Minority Aged. E. Percil Stanford,
    Editor. San Diego, Calif.: Center on Aging, School
    of Social Work, San Diego State University, 1977,
    pp. 41-62.

Poverty, discrimination, segregation and little or no
access to scientific health care providers seem to
have produced a selected body of elderly--perhaps only
the strong survive--because the mortality picture of
very old Blacks (over 75 years) is generally better
than that of their Anglo peers, argues the author.
Nevertheless, for all Black elderly, there is a per-
sistent pattern of higher incidence of most chronic
diseases, days of forced inactivity and visits to physicians. There is very little detailed information
about the relative well-being and health care needs
of Black aged. Studies which lump non-elderly with
elderly are misleading, while studies of Black elderly alone document conditions without offering a yard-
stick for determining the relative severity or frequency of problems for Blacks, states the author. The
author concludes that while sickle-cell has captured
the attention of many Americans, the most severe
health problem of Black elderly, and for the overall

(Weaver, Jerry L.)

community, is hypertension. As early as 1966 it was reported that "in any age group the likelihood of heart disease with hypertension is greater for Blacks than for White persons." Especially threatened are Black women: fully 71 percent of Black women over 50 years of age in a study of New Orleans residents were found to be hypertensive, concludes the writer.

Wilson, James L. "Geriatric Experiences with the Negro Aged." Geriatrics, Vol. 8, February, 1953, pp. 88-92.

The author states that while there are no sharp differences in the majority of diseases affecting the Black aged and those effecting the White race in the same age bracket, there are certain differences in etiologic factors and incidence of ailments which merit consideration and correction. On the basis of a study of an active Negro population between the ages of 55 and 91, the diseases encountered may be listed in the order of their occurrence as: (1) cardiovascular disease, with or without hypertension; (2) arteriosclerosis, generalized; (3) hypertrophic and infectious arthritis and osteoarthritis; (4) calcified fibroma uteri; (5) hypertrophied prostate; (6) carcinoma of breast, uterus and stomach; (7) pneumonia and influenza; (8) diabetes mellitus with complicating infections and gas gangrene; (9) pulmonary tuberculosis; (10) aneurysm; (11) leg ulcers, due to varicose veins, arteriosclerosis, diabetes, trauma or sickle-cell anemia; (12) cirrhosis of the liver; (13) senile dementia, cerebral arteriosclerosis and cataracts; (14) vitiligo; (15) arterio-venous fistula due to trauma; and (16) ainhum. The author points out that the FACTORS determining the incidence of certain ailments in aged Blacks are primarily economic. Where they exist, a low wage scale and long working hours tend to undermine body resistance. Poor housing and overcrowding with attendant unsanitary conditions predispose to infectious diseases. The existence of crowded districts and alleys in cities promotes disease and crime. Trauma encountered in hazardous occupations is responsible for production of certain surgical ailments. Inadequate diet promotes low serum proteins which retard tissue repair. In certain areas some hospitals refuse to admit Blacks who, in many instances, are not hospitalized when necessary. Of nearly equal significance is the refusal of several medical schools to give postgraduate and refresher courses to Black physicians. Not withstanding these economic and educational barriers, the span of life and the total Black population have continued to increase. Scientific investigation serves to stress the need for greater opportunities for the Negro population, especially

(Wilson, James L.)

in economic, educational, health and hospitalization
areas. The writer declares that there are essentially
no major differences between the diseases of the Black
aged and those of the White race in the same age
bracket. Certain diseases, however, have a higher incidence in the Black: hypertensive heart disease, advanced generalized arteriosclerosis and pulmonary tuberculosis. The author concludes that the latter is
on the decline. Incidence of carcinoma, as a whole,
is lower than in the White race, but fibromyoma uteri
is more commonly found. Vitiligo is seen more frequently than in the White race, and the rare finding
of ainhum has not been reported in the White man. Only the latent cases of sickle-cell anemia live to
reach an old age.

Young, John L., et al. "Incidence of Cancer in United
    States Blacks." Cancer Research, Vol. 35, November,
    1975, pp. 3523-3536.

Incidence rates for the Black population of six Standard Metropolitan Statistical Areas in the United
States are examined using data collected in the Third
National Cancer Survey, 1969 to 1971. For all sites
combined, Black males had the highest rates among the
four major race-sex groups; Black females had the lowest rates. For fourteen common sites accounting for
80% of the cancers among Blacks, Black/White ratios,
survival data, trends between 1935 and 1969, and geo-
graphic variation are presented. United States Black
data, adjusted to an African Standard, are compared
with similar data from Nigeria, Rhodesia, and South
Africa. It has been suggested that the high rates
among Black males can be explained by census underenumeration. However, it has shown that, while there was
considerable underenumeration of Black males, aged 20
to 54, there was an overenumeration of Black males
aged 65 and over, state the writers. None of the patterns previously discussed were significantly altered.
Thus, high rates among Black males cannot be explained
on the basis of denominators that were too low, declare
the authors. An analysis of survey data by socioeconomic status is currently being undertaken by the National Cancer Institute utilizing census tract data.
It is hoped that such an analysis will enable the
Black/White differences noted in this report to be
further understood, conclude the authors.

5.   BLACK AGED AND MENTAL HEALTH

Carter, James H.   "Differential Treatment of The Elderly
    Black: Victims of Stereotyping." *Postgraduate
    Medicine*, Vol. 52, November, 1972, pp. 211-214.

The writer discusses two case studies involving elderly Blacks. He points out that aged Black persons, far
from being homogeneous, make up heterogeneous groupings. Dr. Carter argues that many Blacks do not seek
early Social Security or public assistance but instead want gainful employment. He observes that the
generalization that the elderly Black will find gratification outside the world of work seems to be a gross
misunderstanding. The author concludes that with a
view toward correcting past and present mistakes, he
would suggest that a starting point could be an independent cultural education including community involvement, study of pertinent social data, and a hard
honest look on the part of physicians at cultural issues as they relate to the elderly Black.

_____. "A Psychiatric Strategy For Aged Blacks in
The Future." *Proceedings of Black Aged in The Future*.
Jacquelyne J. Jackson, Editor. Durham, N. C.: Center
for the Study of Aging and Human Development, Duke
University, 1973, pp. 94-100.

The author observes that within the past decades psychiatry has made only token efforts to combat racism
and to improve psychiatric care for Black patients,
especially elderly Blacks. He also points out that in
spite of preventive measures, he anticipates that aged
Blacks in the future will be suffering some mental
illness. The writer declares that the White therapist
can be effective with Black patients if he learns to
understand the cultural and social values of Blacks.

_____. "Psychiatry's Insensitivity To Racism and Ag-
ing." *Psychiatric Opinion*, Vol. 10, No. 6, December,
1973, pp. 21-25.

According to Dr. Carter, racism, clearly a mental
health problem, places every Black American in the
position of being "psychologically terrorized, poli-
tically tyrannized, socially minimized and economically ignored." Because of racism, mental health professionals have been guilty of making too many in-
valid generalizations about the Black elderly, with
too little selective research regarding the relevance
of race to aging. Few psychiatrists will deny that
they should carry a special responsibility to combat-
ing racism. Yet most seem hesitant to become personally involved in solving those problems stemming from
racism. Obviously, the "good-will" of psychiatry is

(Carter, James H.)

encouraging, but it does very little to combat racism,
states Dr. Carter. What is actually needed is a personal involvement in attacking racism, which gives
rise to most of the mental health problem of the Black
patient. The Black, elderly psychiatric patient,
whose problems would be expected to be compounded by
age, constitutes a special group of patients who generally defy all of our current "accepted criteria for
treatment." This clearly, according to the author,
indicates that we need to begin to evaluate our traditional methods of treating Black patients. The Black,
elderly patients may be seen as being special in that
they are not only discriminated against because of
age, but because of race. Seemingly, most psychiatrists have found little satisfaction in treating
Black patients, and it would be expected that they
will find still less gratification in taking care of
aged Black patients. Further, the private practice
of psychiatry, which typically treats the middle-class
neurotic patient, is obviously more rewarding finan-
cially than service in public clinics or mental hospitals that treat the aged and the severely mentally
disturbed patient, concludes the author.

_____. "Psychiatry, Racism and Aging." Journal of The
American Geriatrics Society, Vol. 20, No. 7, July,
1972, pp. 343-346.

The basis for present inadequacies in the treatment
of aged Black psychiatric patients is discussed.
Training programs in psychiatry should include working with people of a different race. The philosophi-
cal and social aspects of Black culture should receive more attention. There is often a direct relationship between social status and type of mental illness. Many of the Black patient's problems are related to race, and he is confronted with more obsta-
cles in obtaining appropriate help, argues the author.
For elderly Black people, there is pressing need for
better integration of mental health services with
other health and social services, concludes the author. Dr. Carter states that the nation must eventually develop programs to make it possible for all
Americans to cope, regardless of their race or age.
Without a reasonable amount of research and evaluation, it is possible to go down the wrong road to the
point of no return. It is time that psychiatrists, in
addition to looking at Black pathology, review the
possibilities for relieving system deficiencies, including the impact of racism, concludes the author.

Carter, James H. "Psychiatry, Racism, and Aging." Pro-
    ceedings of The Research Conference on Minority Group
    Aged in The South. Jacquelyne J. Jackson, Editor.
    Durham, N. C.: Center for the Study of Aging and Hu-
    man Development, Duke University Medical Center, 1972,
    pp. 125-130.

Up to the present time, approximately nine out of
every ten psychotic Black patients have been institutionalized and given protective or custodial care instead of active treatment, contends the author. As
for the less severely disturbed, most clinics, finding
traditional therapy ineffective, have been content to
let the Black patient drop away, rather than break
with custom and tradition to develop alternative treatment methods. Effective treatment of Black and lower
income groups seems to require multiple forms of intervention. The author argues that historically there
have been three lines of approach to the treatment of
mental illness--the physical, the psychological and
the social. While all three forms of intervention are
utilized to some extent, at the present time it is
characteristic for Black patients to receive the physical approach (chemical-somatic). Conditions of life
of the Black patient, particularly from low income
families, are such that a simultaneous attack on all
levels is frequently required. The writer points out,
for example, combining active environmental manipula-
tion, such as job modification, with physical thera-
pies, to effect the speediest amelioration of symptoms,
with appropriate forms of psychological intervention.
There is a pressing need to achieve fuller integration
of mental health services with other social, educational, health and welfare services in the community, and
this especially applies to the aged. Families on the
lower socio-economic ladder have a multiplicity of unmet health, economic and social needs. The author
states that it is difficult to see how effective mental health services can be rendered by a community mental health facility which pays no attention to the totality of needs, and which endeavors to dispense phy-
siological prescriptions without regard to the whole
life situation of the patient, concludes Dr. Carter.

Elam, Lloyd C. "Critical Factors For Mental Health in Ag-
    ing Black Populations." Ethnicity, Mental Health and
    Aging. Los Angeles: Gerontology Center, University
    of Southern California, April, 1970, p. 2.

The author surmises that one of the critical factors
for mental health in the Black aged populations is the
proper understanding more and best mental technique
needs to be employed in dealing with this group. Unlike the White aged, the Black elderly have special
problems: they are poorer, had a harder life, in poor
health, and racism is ever present.

Faulkner, Audrey Olsen et al. "Life Strengths and Life
    Stress: Exploration in the Measurement of Mental
    Health of The Black Aged." American Journal of Ortho-
    psychiatry, Vol. 45, January, 1975, pp. 102-110.

    This paper describes an attempt to understand the
    self-concept, social characteristics, personal
    strengths, and frailties of a group of older Black men
    and women in order to tailor mental health and social
    work services to their needs. Difficulties inherent
    in obtaining such information were minimized by a
    methodology that integrated the research and service
    aspects of the project. Results of the pilot study,
    and service implications, are discussed. The results
    show that in spite of a life full of stress and diffi-
    culties, the majority of the Black men and women in
    this group have a highly positive self-concept, com-
    pare themselves favorably with other people their age,
    and express relatively high satisfaction with life and
    themselves, all indices which show their strength, and
    which we consider highly relevant to mental health.
    They do, however, tend to feel victims of their en-
    vironment (which, in view of the very high crime rate
    in the area they live in, is a realistic appraisal)
    and some seem socially isolated in spite of their
    eagerness for contact, conclude the authors.

Hawkins, Brin. "Mental Health and The Black Aged." Men-
    tal Health: A Challenge to the Black Community.
    Lawrence E. Gary, Editor. Philadelphia: Dorrance &
    Co., 1978, pp. 166-178.

    The author discusses the stress factors that affect
    the mental health of the Black Aged. These factors
    include the lack of sufficient income, housing and
    health care. He also states that isolation and lack
    of social contact and communication can be as physi-
    cally debilitating as health dysfunctions and may lead
    directly to emotional stress. The older person who
    has lost family, friends, and satisfying social roles
    may lose the will to eat, to participate, and even-
    tually the will to live. Dr. Hawkins concludes that
    these stresses are compounded for a large number of
    Black elderly who are left without the necessary econ-
    omic and personal resources to maintain an active and
    meaningful social life.

Jackson, Jacquelyne J. "Negro Aged in North Carolina."
    North Carolina Journal of Mental Health, Vol. 4, No.
    1, 1970, pp. 43-52.

    The author points out that, in North Carolina, more
    active intervention by community mental health and
    other agencies in areas of critical social concerns
    must take place. Apparently, too many day centers

(Jackson, Jacquelyne J.)

within the state are yet too much concerned about the
racial identity of the clients whom they will and
will not service, or yield only to token desegrega-
tion. According to the author too few psychiatrists
and others speak up "loud and clear" about such problems, as did too few North Carolinians generally
about the recent events which indicated that some
state workers were receiving wages below the minimum
wage scale--a fact which some persons may interpret
as unrelated, e.g., to Black aged, but which is quite
related inasmuch as, again, we are back to income!
Income affects, in various ways, adjustment in old
age, states Dr. Jackson. Community mental health centers, it seems to the author, might assist further in
helping to deal with such problems as those of pover-
ty--including employment and sufficient income, racism, youth problems and suicides. A resolution of
these types of problems would help to improve considerably the conditions and mental health statuses of
Blacks and of other aged within North Carolina, contends Dr. Jackson. This paper about Black aged in
North Carolina was concerned chiefly with providing
some limited demographic data about such persons; with
pointing out the need for further studies about them,
with especial emphasis upon factors affecting their
mental health statuses; and with suggesting that community mental health centers throughout the state
might--in fact, should--play significant roles in
helping to reduce the types of social conditions
which tend to affect adversely the mental health statuses of Blacks, and of others who are aged, concludes
the author.

Peterson, John and Lillie Thomas. "The Social Psychology
of Black Aging: The Effects of Self-Esteem and Perceived Control on The Adjustment of Older Black
Adults." Health and The Black Aged. Wilbur H. Watson, et al., Editors. Washington, D. C.: National
Center on Black Aged, 1978, pp. 97-104.

The authors point out that the negative attitudes
toward aging and the problem of race accentuates the
problems of aging for older Blacks in the United
States. It seems likely that the pervasive segregation and discrimination experienced by elderly Blacks
may be especially influential in the development of
feelings of low self-esteem and pessimism and result
in psychological withdrawal and physical decline in
old age. In contrast, however, if the older person is
able to maintain personal control and feelings of mas-
tery, he is more likely to experience personal effi-
cacy and positive life satisfaction, argues the writer. In accord with the results of the present study,

(Peterson, John and Lillie Thomas)

it found that the older Blacks reported a substantial
degree of life satisfaction, and interestingly enough,
higher morale than younger Blacks. According to the
authors, although there were significant variations in
life satisfaction scores among members of the sample,
the determinants of these variations were not clear.
They could be attributed to self-esteem, perceived
control, or mediated by the general involvement of the
sample in the adult activity center. However, despite
the limitations of the writer's analyses of the results, it does appear worthwhile that social policies
should be established to change the social environmental effects that may reduce the self-worth and personal responsibility of older Black adults, conclude
the writers.

Polansky, Grace. "Planning for the Specially Disadvantaged
    Minority Groups: Clinical Experience." National
    Conference on Alternatives To Institutional Care For
    Older Americans: Practice and Planning. Eric
    Pfeiffer, Editor. Durham: Center For the Study of
    Aging and Human Development, Duke University Medical
    Center, 1973, pp. 116-121.

The author contends that the older Black comes to the
clinician because he is feeling pain and has grossly
unmet common human needs. Remember that this is relative, that Blacks have the same range as Whites, have
achieved just as satisfying and effective and useful
a level of functioning in many cases; could in all,
given equal opportunity in every sphere for development of individual potential. He may come with hos-
tility, distrust, open or masked, may not want to come
at all, may need more encouragement, a glimmer of hope
that, here, he is going to be treated with dignity un-
threatened, with respect, with his rights of self determination seen as strong as anyone's, states Dr.
Pfeiffer. He may put you on, may continue any of a
variety of responses he's had to learn to survive in
an essentially hostile world. Dependence may have
worked, throttled back expression of true feelings may
have been or seemed necessary. His "security" may
have seemed to him to be within the White, benevolent
world, he tells us. His sense of status is a mirror
image in some cases, reflected. He sees himself as
others see him. Or he may come proudly. The Black who
has lived in the North for decades and returned seems
often to feel more hope, more power, not to be so often caught in the helpless, hopeless, powerless syn-
drome, argues the author. The activism of the largely
younger Blacks may have liberated something in them
too dangerous for many to express openly before; "more
often with the people in our clinical setting it seems

(Polansky, Grace)

to have been frightening, I think, as suppressed rage
stirs, threatens to get out of control, feels dangerous," declares the writer. "There is rage, under-
standably, on some level, and this is where our job
comes in, to help this be a force for constructive
change," concludes the author.

Reynolds, David and Richard A. Kalish. "Anticipation of
Futurity as a Function of Ethnicity and Age." Journal
of Gerontology, Vol. 29, No. 2, March, 1974, pp. 224-
231.

This article is based on a larger study of attitudes
and expectations; 434 residents of Greater Los Angeles,
approximately equally divided by four ethnic and
three age groups, stated how long they wished to live
and how long they expected to live. The authors anticipated that the older persons expected to and wanted
to live longer than the younger age cohorts. The writers were surprised that the Black respondents were
significantly more likely to expect to live and want
to live longer than Japanese Americans, Mexican Americans, and White Americans. The aged Blacks did not
fear death. They concluded that other differences,
such as their sex, between ethnic groups were minimal.

Scott, Judith and Charles M. Gaitz. "Ethnic and Age Differences in Mental Health Measurements." Diseases of
The Nervous Systems, Vol. 36, No. 7, July, 1975, pp.
389-393.

The sample included 1441 respondents stratified by
sex, the three major ethnic groups of Houston--Anglo
(an ethnic designation used commonly in the southwest,
meaning White, non-Mexican-American), Black, and Mex-
ican-American, two family socioeconomic levels (working class and lower-middle class), and six age groups
ranging from a 20-29 age group to a 75-94 group. To
increase the validity of responses, the interviewers
were matched ethnically to the respondents. One hypothesis of the relationships of social stress and
mental illness states that, because of the effects of
racial prejudice, minority groups would suffer more
psychological stress than the dominant ethnic group;
and that the added stress should be reflected in more
psychological-symptom expression. To support such an
hypothesis the authors would predict, for example,
higher mean symptom reports from, first, the Blacks,
secondly, from the Mexican-Americans, and then the
lowest score from the Anglos. Our data, however, show
the opposite. The writers found the highest level of
symptom expression by Anglos, then by Mexican-Americans, and finally the lowest level of symptom expression by Blacks.

Shader, Richard I., and Martha Tracy. "On Being Black,
    Old, and Emotionally Troubled: How Little is Known."
    Psychiatric Opinion, Vol. 10, No. 6, December, 1973,
    pp. 26-32.

This article reviewed multiple factors in pursuing
answers to the questions regarding the identification
and management of elderly Blacks in one well-circum-
scribed, well-covered catchment area. Evaluating all
of the statistics which the authors have gathered,
there are few hard conclusions to be drawn. They service a Black elderly population which is, at the minimum, one percent of our total population. Black elderly patients comprise only 3.7 percent of our geriatric inpatient experience. A significant age difference exists between the writers' elderly White and
Black patients. Although many explanations have been
considered in evaluation of low number of Black geriatric patients, no single explanation appears to account for the very small numbers of elderly Blacks.
The writers declare it is probably that several causes
contribute in varying degree in various communities.
Superimposed on a background of early mortality, these
factors could begin to explain the relatively low frequency of Black geriatric patients seen in our urban
psychiatric facilities, conclude the authors. It
seems very important to them, however, to acknowledge
how little we know, declare the authors.

Solomon, Barbara. "Ethnicity, Mental Health and the Older
    Black Aged." Ethnicity, Mental Health and Aging.
    Gerontology Center, University of Southern California,
    Los Angeles, 1970, pp. 10-13.

The writer points out that the Black aged have special
mental health problems than those of other ethnic
groups. Therefore they need special attention.

Whanger, Alan D. and H. Shan Wang. "Clinical Correlates
    of the Vibratory Sense in Elderly Psychiatric Pa-
    tients." Journal of Gerontology, Vol. 29, No. 1,
    January, 1974, pp. 39-45.

The authors state that the vibratory threshold (VT)
was measured quantitatively at the wrist and knees of
acutely admitted and chronically hospitalized elderly
psychiatric patients and compared with a cohort of elderly persons living in the community. The VT was
markedly elevated in all groups as compared with a
young controlled group. The VT of the psychiatric
patients was significantly higher (hence implying neurologic impairment) than that of the community volunteers. The measurement at the wrists was the more
useful one clinically. The VT of Black subjects was
significantly lower than that of White subjects.

(Whanger, Alan D. and H. Shan Wang)

Those on inadequate diets had a significantly elevated VT, as did those using tobacco, when compared to non-users. Subjects with diabetes, syphilis, and severe organic brain syndromes also had significantly elevated VT, conclude the writers.

6. BLACK AGED AND ECONOMICS

Beattie, Walter M. "The Aging Negro: Some Implications For Social Welfare Services," Phylon, Vol. 21, Summer, 1960, pp. 131-135.

This article is an attempt to raise questions as to whether the patterns of health, welfare and leisure-time services which emerging for our aging population throughout the United States have relevance or meaning for the aging Black and his family. It is essential that this question be raised, especially as one considers the fact that the greater part of our planning for such services is taking place in metropolitan centers where the population is comprised of a significant proportion of Blacks, contends the author. In addition, those areas of the city known sociologically as the "zones of transition" are increasingly becoming the place of residence for the aged, both White and Black as well as for the Black population of all ages. We must be constantly aware of individual differences in carrying out our responsibilities of planning for all older persons, states Beattie. The writer surmises, however, in our concern over the individuality of all older persons, we must also give recognition to the racial and socio-economic differences between those groups of persons who comprise our older population. The author declares if we can do this through the development of more basic knowledge as to the composition of our aged population, we will begin to go a long way toward meeting people where they are and in helping them to achieve the utmost for which their capacities allow. He concludes if we do not, we will be creating community programs for older persons in the image of those groups and interests with which we may have the most acquaintance. This, certainly, is a bias which social welfare programs must avoid if they are to truly relate to the interests and concerns of all older persons in each of our communities, continues the author.

Davis, Donald L. "Growing Old Black." Employment Prospects of Aged Blacks, Chicanos, and Indians. Washington, D. C.: National Council on The Aging, 1971, pp. 27-51.

The author points out that as Blacks grow old they have little to look forward to. In many cases Blacks

(Davis, Donald L.)

have to continue to work after they reach retirement age because they can not make ends meet on their Social Security Benefits.

Davis, Frank G.   "The Impact of Social Security Taxes Upon The Poor: The Cases of the Black Community."   Economics of Aging. Ann Arbor: Institute of Gerontology, University of Michigan-Wayne State University, 1976, pp. 41-53.

The author states that the Black community suffers most from Social Security Taxes because many Blacks die before they can receive Social Security benefits. Moreover, most Blacks can not afford increases in Social Security tax because they have a lower income than Whites; therefore, their take home pay checks are smaller.

Gillespie, Bonnie J.   "Elderly Blacks and The Economy." Journal of Afro-American Issues, Vol. 3, Summer/Fall, 1975, pp. 324-335.

This paper briefly outlines the general situation of the elderly Black, the present economy, and the interaction effect. The author states that there are approximately 1.7 million elderly Black. They live in all parts of the country, but about 3/5 of them live in the South and most tend to live in urban areas in the South. Dr. Gillespie points out that the disproportionate distribution of income sources by total aggregate incomes, as well as by percent of families receiving incomes of specified types, indicate a considerable need for revising sources of both higher dependable and increased incomes for aged Blacks. He concludes that as long as racism abounds in America the problems of Black elders will continue to be acute. When we attack racism and its institutionalization we assist in bringing about the economic or material and psychological well-being or quality of life of the elderly Black.

Henderson, George.   "The Negro Recipient of Old-Age Assistance: Results of Discrimination." Social Casework, Vol. 46, 1965, pp. 208-214.

This article is based on an exploratory study of 100 aged Blacks who were recipients of Old-Age Assistance grants in Detroit, Michigan. The main purpose of this article was to examine some of the problems peculiar to aged Blacks. The writer argues that racial discrimination is the cause of many of the problems of today's (1965) aged Blacks, and until it is eliminated, we shall merely be attacking effects, not causes.

(Henderson, George)

He surmises that today's aged Black is different from today's aged White because he is "Black" by society's definition, with its socioeconomic consequences. Mr. Henderson suggests that this is his uniqueness, and this alone should be an adequate basis for compensatory treatment. For he has, indeed, been played in double jeopardy; first, by being Black, and second, by being old. The author concludes that it is safe to predict that with a continued racial discrimination, there will be an increasing number of aged Blacks living on public assistance programs.

Hudson, Gossie Harold. "Social and Economic Problems Facing the Black Elderly." Share, Vol. 3, No. 2, (Black Educators' Council For Human Sciences, North Carolina A & T State University), January 7, 1975, pp. 1-6.

The title tells what this article is about. The writer states that psychological damages help to compound the problems of social and economic insecurity. Dr. Hudson contends that there is a need for more research in the area of Black gerontology by students as well as scholars of history.

Oliver, Mamie O. "Elderly Blacks and The Economy." Journal of Afro-American Issues, Vol. 3, Summer/Fall 1975, pp. 316-323.

The writer argues that elderly Black Americans experience a vital balance or survival quotient resulting from a blend of strategy, inner integrity, "style," pride and positive spirit. Despite group suppression, rampant racism, racial exploitation, second class citizenship, psychological "trips" focused on despair, physical weakness (hypertension, etc.), old age is a considerable achievement for many elderly Black Americans. The author states it could be said that stress, in this instance, produces with the years, fervor, inner growth, and courage. The elderly Black American, this writer submits, is the possessor of integrity and balance and is capable of defending the dignity of his own life style against all physical and economic threats. Oliver concludes the Black elderly knows solidarity in the midst of racial prejudice, low economic status, and personal suffering, a commitment to justice for ALL mankind. All this should serve to challenge the Black family in America and other youngsters and oldsters to take and pursue life--it is the opportunity and blessing afforded all mundane humans, states Oliver.

Palm, Charles H.   "The Future of The Black Aged In Ameri-
     ca." Proceedings of Black Aged in The Future. Jac-
     quelyne J. Jackson, Editor. Durham, N. C.: Center for
     the Study of Aging and Human Development, Duke Univer-
     sity, 1973, pp. 86-93.

     The author asserts that the future of the Black Aged
     in America ultimately depends upon the emergence of
     human values as being the primary focus, a redeploy-
     ment of our federal, state and county resources, re-
     ordering of our priorities and the motivation to seek
     solutions for our numerous problems by means of a hor-
     izontal approach in lieu of a simplistic vertical or
     linear approach. He concludes that the problem of the
     Black Aged in America is an extension of the problem
     of the Aged in America in general and more particular-
     ly an extension of the problem of the economically de-
     prived aged in a culture which focuses on youth and
     which frequently attempts to solve its problems by for-
     mulas, slogans and cliches.

7.   BLACK AGED AND HOUSING

Isserman, Abraham J.   "Housing For The Aged Blacks." Pro-
     ceedings of Black Aged in The Future. Jacquelyne J.
     Jackson, Editor. Durham, N. C.: Center for The Study
     of Aging and Human Development, Duke University, 1973,
     pp. 34-49.

     The writer points out that housing for Blacks and for
     the elderly Blacks has been blocked by The Department
     of Housing and Urban Development's rules and regula-
     tions. He gives fourteen housing needs of the Black
     elderly. These needs are applicable in most part to
     all elderly persons. Mr. Isserman concludes that to
     fulfill these needs will require strong dedication and
     intensive work in building coalitions of all people
     and organizations of good-will determined to put Amer-
     ica back on a course where its resources will be de-
     voted to the well-being of the people of this country.

Jackson, Hobart C.   "Housing and Geriatric Centers For Ag-
     ing and Aged Blacks." Proceedings of Black Aged in
     The Future. Jacquelyne J. Jackson, Editor. Durham,
     N. C.: Center for The Study of Aging and Human Devel-
     opment, Duke University, 1973, pp. 23-33.

     The author feels that there are general inadequacies
     in our social institutions and specific housing inad-
     equacies for aged Blacks. Because of this, he recom-
     mended very strongly that a movement be undertaken for
     the development of geriatric centers in Black communi-
     ties. He concludes that a redistribution of income is
     vital if the Black elderly are to be removed from the
     kind of grinding poverty that no one was meant to

(Jackson, Hobart C.)

endure. Jackson continued to surmise that the implementation of a goal of power for the powerless would
give the minority elderly the priority position they
deserve.

Jackson, Jacquelyne J. "Social Impact of Housing Relocation Upon Urban, Low-Income Black Aged." Gerontologist, Vol. 12, Spring, 1972, pp. 32-37.

The author did a comparison of successful and non-
successful Black aged applicants for a public, age-
segregated housing complex in Durham, North Carolina
to determine characteristics favoring acceptability.
Those whose objective characteristics (e.g. being male
and married) more nearly approximated dominant social
patterns and whose subjective characteristics (e.g.
dependency) tended to conform to traditional stereotypes of Blacks gained admission more often than those
rejected. One significant social impact, in the mi-
crocosm, is that of the social consequences of such
discriminatory selectivity among Blacks only. One
major implication of the study is an apparent tenden-
cy for the selection processes to favor those among
the Blacks who, in some sense, may be the least de-
prived. In other words, here as in other areas involving younger and older Blacks, those "who get in"
are those who tend, on the one hand, to approximate
more nearly those objective characteristics (such as
being male, younger, or married) favored by the larger society, and, on the other hand, who display subjective characteristics not favored by the larger
society, except as they may be found within minority
groups (such as dependency), argues Dr. Jackson.
Hence, this study suggests, anew, serious considerations of the consequences of selectivity outward of
the "best," and rejection of the "rest" of the Blacks,
whether it be in housing for the aged, education for
the youth or employment for the adults, concludes the
writer.

Stretch, John J. "Are Aged Blacks Who Manifest Difference
in Community Security Also Different in Coping Reactions?" Aging and Human Development, Vol. 7, 1976,
pp. 171-184.

This article was based on seventy-two aged Blacks,
equally divided between those residing in a high-rise
public housing project and those living in the community awaiting admission. They were interviewed to test
the theory that differences in community security
would predict differences in coping reactions. Data
on perceived community security and reported medical,
social and mental coping reactions were collected,

(Stretch, John J.)

using a simply and directly worded, precoded, stimu-
lus-response instrument developed by the author. Respondents were assigned to either a high or to a low
community security group by two methods: first, they
were assigned a place of residence; next they were
assigned according to their obtained community security score. The author concludes that the results in
general supported the theory. Of the two empirical
indicators of community security, however, larger differences in coping reaction scores were found in the
high scoring and low scoring community security groups
than in the high-rise and community groups.

8. BLACK AGED AND RELIGION

Jericho, Bonnie J. "Longitudinal Changes in Religious
     Activity Subscores of Aged Blacks." Black Aging,
     Vol. 2, Nos. 4-6, April, June and August, 1977, pp.
     17-24.

This presentation is primarily concerned with the tem-
poral stability of religious activity subscores among
aged Blacks, as well as with factors, including religious attitude subscores, which may affect that stability. Using secondary data from the Duke University
Longitudinal Study, it has three specific purposes.
The first is an examination by sex of the longitudinal
stability of the religious activity subscores of the
Blacks in both Rounds 1 and 3 of the Duke study. The
second is the isolation of some of the variables affecting the stability of those subscores over time.
The third is a discussion of certain gerontological
and religious implications of the findings. The study
of change in the stability of the religious activity
subscores of aged Blacks between roughly the years
1955 and 1965 showed no consistent decrease with increasing age among them. The stability of their religious activities was affected by socioeconomic status.
In general, the lower the socioeconomic status the
greater the decrease in religious activities. This
phenomenon probably occurred because aged Blacks of
lower socioeconomic status compensate for their reduced church attendance with increased reading of religious literature and other types of compensatory
activities measured by the religious activity scale,
argues the author. This would also suggest that the
study is historically bound, states Jericho. The percentage of lower socioeconomic aged Blacks who would
have access to a television and available means of
transportation in 1955 to 1965 would have increased by
1977 and such factors would not affect the religious
activity subscore in the same way. The author concludes that perhaps the most important gerontological

(Jericho, Bonnie J.)

implications of this study are (1) the need for the
development of a more sophisticated instrument to measure longitudinal changes in religious patterns among
older persons; and (2) the need for a carefully designed and self-executed study of religious patterns
among older Blacks. Such a study contains a sufficiently large number of Blacks, so as to permit cross-
variable comparisons of a meaningful nature. According to the writer, one of the current problems in the
gerontological literature concerning Blacks is the insufficient sampling of Blacks makes it almost impos-
sible to obtain valid findings about them. Particularly worthy of investigation are the effects of socioeconomic status (including sex) and widowhood upon
religious activities and attitudes in the later years.
Theorists in the area of religion and aging should de-
vote more attention to the effects of socioeconomic
status upon religious activities and attitudes of elderly people as they continue to age, as well as to
the prior effects of socioeconomic status upon the religious activities and attitudes which accompany them
into old age, argues the writer.

Smith, Earl. "Two Brothers: 100 Years of Caring." Jet,
     October 10, 1974, pp. 22-23.

     Article discusses Albert Peters, who is 102 years old,
     and his brother Paul Peters, who is 94 years old and
     blind. Albert takes care of his brother and has been
     doing so for nearly most of his adult life. Both are
     deeply religious men and are regularly churchgoers.

Walker, Bishop John. "How Organized Religion Can and
     Should Meet The Needs of Aged Blacks." Action For
     Aged Blacks: When? A Conference of The National Cau-
     cus on The Black Aged. Jacquelyne J. Jackson, Editor.
     Washington, D. C.: National Caucus on The Black Aged,
     1973, pp. 52-54.

     The writer surmises that the whole question of a minis-
     try to the aging is one which has traditionally been
     within the Church's realm and sphere of activity. He
     asserts that the organized churches of America, be they
     Christian or non-Christian, will combine their re-
     sources and work together to develop communities that
     are rich and fulfilling for the young and old alike.
     The Bishop concludes that the young need the aging, as
     the aging need the young. Together they can develop
     creative programs and creative life styles for all our
     people.

9.   BLACK AGED POPULATION

Dowd, James J. et al.   "Aging in Minority Populations: An
    Examination of The Double Jeopardy Hypothesis."
    Journal of Gerontology, Vol. 33, 1978, pp. 427-435.

    Utilizing data from a large (N=1269) multistage proba-
    bility sample of middle-aged and aged Blacks, Mexican
    Americans and Anglos living in Los Angeles County, in-
    dicators of relative status and primary group inter-
    action, were analyzed to determine the degree and na-
    ture of any ethnic variation. It was found that dif-
    ferences among the three ethnic groups do exist in
    some cases, particularly on income and self-assessed
    health, constitute a case of double jeopardy for the
    minority aged. But while double jeopardy was found
    to be an accurate characterization of the Black and
    Mexican American aged on several variables, the data
    also suggest that age exerts a leveling influence on
    some ethnic variation over time. Variables such as
    frequency of interaction with relatives as well as,
    for Black respondents, the life satisfaction factors
    of Tranquility and Optimism all evidence a certain de-
    cline in the extent of ethnic variation across age
    strata.

Ehrlich, Ira F.   "Toward A Social Profile of The Aged
    Black Population in The United States: An Exploratory
    Study." Aging and Human Development, Vol. 4, Nov. 3,
    1973, pp. 271-276.

    This article is based on a stratified random sample of
    Black men and women aged 70 and over. This study was
    developed in two high rise age segregated urban hous-
    ing units in St. Louis. Normative activity was clas-
    sified in terms of three life styles: alone, recipro-
    cal and nonreciprocal. An internal comparison was
    made with a Black sample and an external comparison
    with a White sample differing on several major demo-
    graphic characteristics. Although the modal activity
    pattern was to do things alone, the findings were
    equivocal with respect to the disengagement framework.
    Involvement with others tended to increase with age,
    and was usually of a religious or leisure time nature.
    Findings of this study suggest the desirability for
    encouraging flexible life style options. The author
    concludes that his study suggested a nonhomogeneous
    sample--particularly in relation to such variables as
    age, income, health and education. Marital status was
    suggested as a variable that may account for signifi-
    cant racial differences.

Smith, T. Lynn.   "The Changing Number and Distribution of
    the Aged Negro Population of the U.S." Phylon, Vol.
    18, 4th Quarter, 1957, pp. 339-354.

The writer asserts that the first half of the Twentieth Century the number of Blacks aged sixty-five
and over increased by 229 percent whereas Blacks of
all ages gained only 70 percent. Even so, however,
the aging of the Black population was less rapid than
that of the total population, for comparable figures
for the latter are almost 300 percent for the aged
contingent and just under 100 percent for those of all
ages, declares Smith. In 1900 only one Black out of
every thirty-four had passed the sixty-fifth birthday,
whereas by 1950 the comparable ratio was one out of
every eighteen. He argues that there will probably be
about 1,150,000 Blacks aged sixty-five and over in
1960, and the number will probably continue to rise
until 1990. A slight decrease in absolute numbers is
likely to take place before the census of the year
2,000. Unless one can forecast the numbers of future
births, the proportions of the aged in future years
cannot be forecast with any degree of accuracy, argues
Smith. The author concludes that it seems unlikely
that the proportions of the aged among Blacks will
equal that among Whites prior to the year 2,000.

10.   RURAL BLACK AGED

Blake, J. Herman. "'Doctor Can't Do Me No Good': Social
    Concomitants of Health Care Attitudes and Practices
    Among Elderly Blacks in Isolated Rural Populations."
    Health and The Black Aged. Wilbur H. Watson, et al.,
    Editors. Washington, D. C.: National Center on
    Black Aged, 1978, pp. 55-62.

The author surmises that practitioners must recognize
that, frequently, there are major gaps between their
expectations and the ability of the elderly to appropriately respond. He found repeated instances of
people being given prescriptions or other instructions
when they were unable to read. Many of the people
have not spent a day in school. Many were functionally illiterate even if they had attended and, as a
consequence, the patients would often end up either
following instructions improperly or not at all. In
either case, medication often produced no improvement
and thus confirmed the belief that "The doctor can't
do me no good." As we attempt to extend the benefits
of health care to the Black elderly we must always
bear in mind that rural residents born 1910 came to
their adulthood in a society very different from the
one we now take for granted, argues the author. To
the extent that their lives still reflect the conditions and experiences of a much earlier generation,

(Blake, J. Herman)

their beliefs and practices will also reflect those
conditions. If we would truly do them any good, we
must "listen eloquently" to their experiences, and respond with sensitivity and understanding, concludes
the author.

Bourg, Carroll J. "A Social Profile of Black Aged in A
   Southern Metropolitan Area." Proceedings of The Re-
   search Conference on Minority Group Aged in the South.
   Jacquelyne J. Jackson, Editor. Durham, N. C.: Center
   for the Study of Aging and Human Development, Duke
   University Medical Center, 1972, pp. 97-106.

The author argues that in household or family composition he found that the extended family remains an un-
explored notion. He contends we are without adequate
terms to identify the various arrangements which have
been arrived at among Black elderly. In addition, it
is characteristic of Black elderly, in contrast to
White elderly, that the presence of adult children or
other relatives in the household usually means that
they have been brought into the homes of the elderly
person(s). If we limit ourselves and government programs to the now accepted identifications of households, heads of household and so on, we exclude large
numbers of Black elderly who can make do and even make
do well in households that combine various persons
all cooperating to the maintenance of the home, argues
Bourg. If the supplementary assistances of govern-
mental agencies can be directed to the actual situations, much can be done to fortify the manifest
strengths of the Black elderly, even though they have
been persons living in a southern metropolitan area,
concludes the writer.

Jackson, Jacquelyne J. "Aged Negroes: Their Cultural De-
   partures From Statistical Stereotypes And Rural-Urban
   Differences." Research Planning and Action for The
   Elderly: The Power and Potential of Social Sciences.
   Donald P. Kent, et al., Editors. New York: Behavior-
   al Publications, Inc., 1972, pp. 501-513.

The major purposes of this article were those of suggesting some areas where aged Blacks tend to become
"cultural departurers" from statistical stereotypes,
and of also suggesting certain variables which may be
useful in distinguishing between rural and urban aged
Blacks. Essentially, both tasks were only partially
successful, due to the scarcity of available data
about aged Blacks, and, no doubt, to the value judgments which the author has imposed upon those data.
Given those limitations, however, Black aged tend to
depart from such statistical stereotypes as those

(Jackson, Jacquelyne J.)

which hold that their marital statuses are significantly different from those of White aged; that their
life expectancies are typically less than those of
Whites (they may be longer at the later age periods);
that they differ significantly from Whites by importance placed upon their families, or that they are
more religious, in poorer health, or less active in
formal organizations than Whites. Some variables
which may be useful in distinguishing between rural
and urban Black aged in southern areas, at least, include those of income sources, material possessions,
health, family, and household factors, friendship and
social contact, church attendance and participation in
church-related organizations, and attitudes toward the
desirability of homes for the aged and toward death,
declares the author. According to the writer, age-
eligibility requirements for Blacks to receive retirement and other old age benefits must be reduced. It
is also necessary for various local, county, and state
governments to become more concerned about, and more
actively involved in programs, planning, and evaluation for Black aged, states the writer. Dr. Jackson
concludes that social gerontologists and practitioners
utilizing their findings have such responsibilities as
those of enhancing the validity and reliability of
statistical stereotypes about Black aged, and of working among and for Black aged to eliminate those valid
stereotypes which are undesirable, and of augmenting
those which are desirable.

Jackson, Jacquelyne J. and A. Davis. "Characteristic Pat-
terns of Aged, Rural Negroes in Macon County." A
Survey of Selected Socioeconomic Characteristics of
Macon County. B. C. Johnson, Editor. Tuskegee, Ala.:
Macon County Community Action Office, 1966.

The title tells what this work is about. The authors
point out that the Black aged in Macon County, Alabama were at the bottom of the social and economic
ladder. They surmise that the various social agencies
in the county showed no real interest in meeting the
pressing needs of Black senior citizens.

Rubenstein, Daniel I. "Social Participation of Aged
Blacks: A National Sample." Proceedings of The Re-
search Conference on Minority Groups Aged in the
South. Jacquelyne J. Jackson, Editor. Durham, N. C.:
Center for the Study of Aging and Human Development,
Duke University Medical Center, 1972, pp. 48-62.

This study found that more of the White elderly lived
alone than did the Black elderly. Moreover, twice as
many White and Black elderly lived in households

(Rubenstein, Daniel I.)

consisting solely of respondent and spouse (presumably husband and wife), states the author. In addition, more Whites than Blacks were found living with a spouse in households containing others. However, examination of larger households showed that the Black elderly lived with more people in their households than did the Whites. Contrary to the stereotype of separated, broken, discontinued families among the Blacks, it was found that only four out of ten Black elderly did so. This family belonging was further evidenced by the finding that more than twice as many Blacks than Whites would be found in companionship households. Intergenerational continuity in households was also found more prevalent for Blacks than for Whites: the Black elderly were more than three times as likely to live in households with grandchildren than were White elderly, according to the author.

"The 130 Year Old Man." Newsweek, October 2, 1972, p. 74.

This article discusses Charlie Smith, an ex-slave, who was thought to be (in 1972) the "oldest" man in the United States. He lived in Bartow, Florida and ran (in 1972) a candy and soft-drink store. Smith outlived three wives. He had a quick sense of humor, a desire to keep active and a firm belief in God. "I ain't so perfect," says Charlie Smith, "but I do try to live nearer to the Commandments."

11.   URBAN BLACK AGED

Barg, Sylvia K. and Carl Hirsch. "A Successor Model For Community Support of Low-Income Minority Group Aged." Aging and Human Development, Vol. 3, 1972, pp. 243-252.

The authors argue that experience in research and community outreach work with low-income urban aged led to the development of a multifocal program approach. The program approach includes case referral and advocacy work with the target population as well as the organization of neighborhood-based groups of elderly residents. The two approaches are intended to achieve both treatment of extant social symptoms of age discrimination and social and political power by the aged to eliminate discrimination on the basis of age. The two approaches provide mutual reinforcement for the success of each, and are based on tenets of social interaction theory as well as an analysis of the social and political powerlessness of the aged in the Model Cities Neighborhood of Philadelphia. The writers conclude that experience in the Model Cities Senior Wheels East has led to considerations involving cross-

(Barg, Sylvia K. and Carl Hirsch)

generational ties between worker and client to
achieve senior power, the role of indigenous community
workers in social welfare agencies working with the
aged as well as the successful application of the approach to the Black, Puerto Rican, and foreign-born
White aged residing in the area.

Clemente, Frank, et al. "Race and Morale of the Urban
    Aged." Gerontologist, Vol. 14, August, 1974, pp. 342-
    344.

Racial differences in morale were analyzed in this
article for comparable samples of 721 Black and 211
White residents of Philadelphia age 65 and over. The
authors argue that a hypothesis suggesting Blacks
have lower morale than Whites was derived from the
literature and tested by regression analysis. The
standardized partial regression coefficient was of
negligible magnitude, and the hypothesis was rejected.
They conclude that possible reasons for the failure
of race to emerge as even a moderate predictor of
morale include Messer's (1968) argument that elderly
Blacks view old age as a reward in itself and McCar-
thy and Yancey's (1971) contention that presumed
racial differences in morale have received little
actual empirical support.

Craig, Dorothy. "Aged Blacks: The Story of Cleveland,
    Ohio." Action For Aged Blacks: When? : A Con-
    ference of The National Caucus on The Black Aged.
    Jacquelyne J. Jackson, Editor. Washington, D. C.:
    National Caucus on The Aged, 1973, pp. 27-31.

The writer discusses senior citizen programs in Cleveland, Ohio, beginning with the organization "Outreach." She also points out that there are 20,000,000
Americans over age 65 (for the year 1973) and a quarter of them live in poverty. Craig acknowledges that
almost half of all older Americans did not complete
elementary school while little more than 1,000,000
are college graduates; and 3,000,000 older people are
considered functionally illiterate. She concludes
that while the picture may be grim for older people,
it does not have to be. With some understanding, effort, and friendliness from the rest of society, the
elderly can be made to feel useful and wanted, concludes the author.

Hearn, H. L. "Career and Leisure Patterns of Middle Aged
    Urban Black." Gerontologist, Vol. 11, Winter, 1971,
    pp. 21-26.

The lack of formal education and opportunities generally have been a tremendous handicap to the aged

(Hearn, H. L.)

Black in America. From the author's research on the
aging artist it was found that second careers which
impart meaning, prestige, and supplement income in
the later years are a source of satisfaction and positive self feelings to those so engaged. The author
concludes that if the aging Black American views his
work as a necessary evil which entails little self-
involvement, perhaps a second career, which could
start at almost any time, will lend more satisfaction
to his retirement years, combining, as it can, "leisure activity" with income supplementation.

Jackson, James S. et al. "Life Satisfaction Among Black
     Urban Elderly." Aging and Human Development, Vol. 8,
     1977-78, pp. 169-179.

This article was based on a sample of 102 Black retired adults residing in noninstitutionalized settings.
The sample was purposely selected from predominantly
Black older adult centers located in the Detroit metropolitan area. Individuals in the sample ranged from
fifty-four to eighty-three years of age with a mean
of 69.5 years. Females comprised 71.6 of the persons
interviewed and were over-represented based upon the
1973 census estimates for this population. In addition to the racial homogeneity of the respondents,
80.9 percent reported a high school education or less.
Reported annual income for the majority of the sample
(87%) was less than three thousand dollars. A large
proportion (62.6%) of the respondents were born and
raised in the South. The authors conclude that their
findings, when viewed in the context of the societal
barriers which perpetually confront Blacks across the
life span, suggest that adjustment to aging, particularly psychologically, might be a different and perhaps relatively easier task in comparison to the adjustment of White majority individuals.

12. BLACK AGED AND NURSING HOMES

Gibbs, Eddie. "Nursing Home Action." Action For Aged
     Blacks: When?: A Conference of The National Caucus
     on The Black Aged. Jacquelyne J. Jackson, Editor.
     Washington, D. C.: National Caucus on The Black Aged,
     1973, pp. 55-57.

The writer declares that the majority of the people in
nursing homes today (1973) are aged people--the aged
Blacks, or what we believe to be the poorest of works
against aged Blacks. Blacks also need to own and
operate their own nursing homes, argues Gibbs. He
concludes that Black people should become more and
more involved, in every way, in trying to improve the
nursing home for the Black aged.

Jackson, Hobart C. "Overcoming Racial Barriers in Senior
    Centers." National Conference on Senior Centers,
    Vol. 2, 1965, pp. 20-28.

The writer points out that for the most part, the
Black aged are treated very poorly in senior centers.
This is due to some degree on the part of the staff
and their racial attitudes and lack of proper training. The aged Black in these centers usually is
alone and without family and friends and has little
personal contact with others in the centers.

Solomon, Barbara. "Social and Protective Services." Work-
    shop on Community Services and The Black Elderly.
    Richard H. Davis, Editor. Los Angeles: Andrus Geron-
    tology Center, University of Southern California,
    1972, pp. 1-11.

The author contends that many Black older people are
in institutional settings in nursing homes, state mental hospitals or what have you because of the lack of
services in the community to support them and allow
them to remain independent in the community. She argues that Black professionals should start to work
hand in hand with the Black residents in the community.

Woolf, Leon M. "Serving Minority Persons in A Senior Cen-
    ter." Challenges Facing Senior Centers in The Nine-
    teen Seventies. Alice G. Wolfson, Editor. New York:
    National Council On The Aging, 1969, pp. 146-152.

The author discusses the Metropolitan Senior Citizens
Center of Baltimore, Maryland. He declares that when
we talk about serving minority persons in senior centers, we almost always think in terms of racial and
religious minorities, particularly Blacks. The author submits that there are growing numbers of aged
persons belonging to other minorities, unrelated to
race or religion, whom we must learn to attract and
serve. He cites a few examples. There are retired
professional people, physically handicapped people,
people with advanced educational backgrounds, poverty-
striken individuals, retired business executives, and
men in general. He asks the question, Is the concept
of the multipurpose senior center broad enough and secure enough to encompass and serve an increasingly
multifaceted clientele?

13.   BLACK AGED AND SUPPORT SERVICES

Anderson, Peggye.   "Support Services and Aged Blacks."
    Black Aging, Vol. 3, No. 3, February, 1978, pp. 53-59.

Although aged Blacks and other groups of elderly people seek and expect support from their families, the
findings in this article reveal that older Blacks frequently underutilize resources in the community. However, in many instances the elderly and their families
need the support of community resources to reduce the
potential and actual strain families experience as a
result of caring for and/or supporting aged family
members, suggests the author. The writer asks a crucial question at this point: "How do we maximize on
the resources available to older people?" If we consider family members as resources for the aged, we can
better design programs to help them assist the elderly,
argues the writer. Such programs can take the form of
intergenerational workshops so that elderly parents
and their adult children can better understand one
another through sharing experiences with other families in similar situations. Day care facilities for
older people, which are slowly appearing in our society, could also eliminate or delay institutionalization and could give adult children free time to pursue
their interests and goals. Another resource that
could be further utilized in the Black community to
support the elderly and their families is the church.
Traditionally, the Black church has been, and is, to
a less extent today, the focal point of social interaction in the Black community, states the author. The
Black church has also been the major vehicle through
which the needs of the elderly are addressed. Therefore, we need to place more emphasis on the use of the
Black church in providing services and dissemination
of information about services that are available to
the elderly in our communities, concludes the author.
The author surmises that in pursuing this research further, we need to tap more services and support mechanisms of the elderly. Therefore, we can better understand the major roles or functions that the family
plays in providing support to aged Blacks. Also, further research can help us assess the extent to which
the society itself fails to provide support to aged
Blacks or if aged Blacks voluntarily do not seek support from the community, states Anderson.

Jackson, Hobart C. "Easing The Plights of The Black Elder-
    ly." Perspectives on Aging, Vol. 4, 1975, pp. 21-22.

The writer contends that the only way to ease the
plights of the Black aged is for local, state, and
federal governments to have effective programs to meet
their needs. These needs include better housing, more

(Jackson, Hobart C.)

income and better social services and health facilities.

Jackson, Jacquelyne J. "Compensatory Care for the Black
    Aged." Minority Aged in America. Occasional papers
    in Gerontology, University of Michigan-Wayne State
    University, 1973.

The writer states that more compensatory care needs to
be devoted to the Black aged because they suffer more
economically than most other elderly. She also contends that more attention should be devoted to the
particular problems of the Black elderly.

Kent, Donald P. et al. "Indigenous Workers As A Crucial
    Link In The Total Support System For Low-Income, Minority Group Aged: A Report Of An Innovative Field
    Technique in Survey Research." Aging and Human Development, Vol. 2, August, 1971, pp. 189-196.

This article traces the development of a concept of
involvement of indigenous workers of all age grades in
work with the low income, minority group aged from its
inception in a survey research context. Employment of
indigenous workers as research interviewers contributed to the lessening of distance between respondents
and interviewers that was, in turn, necessary if appropriate data was to be secured. Problem referral
work in the research context led the authors to investigate broader areas in which the communication
skills and community commitment of the indigenous
worker could be brought to bear in fostering social
change to alleviate the deprivation of low income, minority aged as a group. Recognition is given to problems of maintaining the unique contribution of the indigenous worker when his role becomes institutionalized in establishment agencies.

14. BLACK AGED AND PROFESSIONAL TRAINING

Jackson, Jacquelyne J. "Education and Training Priorities
    For Ethnic Groups." Conferences On The Role of Institutions of Higher Learning in The Study of Aging,
    1972. Richard H. Davis et al., Editors. Los Angeles:
    Ethel Percy Andrus Gerontology Center, University of
    South California, 1973, pp. 131-132.

The author points out that at this conference recommendations were made in four areas: The structure of
problem-solving groups; allocation of federal funds;
priorities for training Blacks; and the content of
training programs. (a) Problem-solving groups, it was
suggested, should organize themselves separately

(Jackson, Jacquelyne J.)

according to type of minority. Then they may join to
solve their common problems. (b) It was felt that
substantial money should be allocated each minority
group at least in proportion to its representation
in the population. The attitude of the National Caucus on the Black Aged is that 12% of federal funding
for aging and the aged should be allocated the Black
aged. Each minority group should decide how the money
will be used. (c) Initial priorities for training
Blacks were articulated. Professionals and paraprofessionals will be prepared to be decision-makers in
various categories such as medicine, economics, law,
and the clergy. Once these persons are trained as
professionals with input into the decision-making
structure, they in turn will train the less educated,
who may then support the interests of the group. (d)
One component to the content of training programs, it
was felt, should be political education for participation in the system. One member of the workshop felt
that content should include teaching ways to solve the
problems of all older persons, regardless of race or
ethnicity.

_____. "Social Stratification of Aged Blacks and Im-
plications For Training Professionals." Proceedings
of Black Aged in The Future. Durham, N. C.: Center
for The Study of Aging and Human Development, Duke
University, 1973, pp. 114-132.

The author is primarily concerned with specifying some
aspects of social similarities and differences among
aged Blacks, and relating those data to existing or
desired training and curricular needs. The most important conclusions, contends Dr. Jackson, are the
diversification of aging and aged Blacks, and the need
to increase substantially adequate knowledge and understanding of aged Blacks, Black aging professionals,
and the future.

Reed, John. "Prospects For Developing Gerontological Train-
ing Programs At Black Institutions." Proceedings of
The Research Conference on Minority Group Aged in the
South. Jacquelyne J. Jackson, Editor. Center for the
Study of Aging and Human Development, Duke University
Medical Center, 1972, pp. 145-147.

The writer contends that many Southern legislatures
have not yet recognized as a problem those who are
Black and aged and needy. Most Blacks, in fact, never
live long enough to become aged problems in the South--
or elsewhere for that matter, argues Reed. The 1970
census data show us that the proportion of persons 65
or more years of age in the Black population is higher

(Reed, John)

than it was in 1960, states the author. Yet, the
Black population in 1970 is younger than it was in
1960. The recognition that Blacks have a sizeable
population 65 or more years of age has not yet come in
many quarters. In fact, we have a sizeable healthy,
aged population, suggests the writer. When the Whites
recognize that a crucial area of research and training
may fall within the realm of ascertaining significant
information about the relatively good health of most
aged Blacks, only then may we get such programs--and
only after they have been instituted in White institutions, concludes the author.

Smith, Stanley H. "The Developing Gerontological Training
Program At Fisk University." Proceedings of The Re-
search Conference on Minority Group Aged in the South.
Jacquelyne J. Jackson, Editor. Durham, N. C.: Center
for The Study of Aging and Human Development, Duke
University Medical Center, 1972, pp. 139-142.

The author believes that in its total configurational
thrust, a graduate program in social gerontology at a
school such as Fisk University should not be similar
in its totality to a graduate program in gerontology
at the University of North Carolina or the University
of Michigan. It should be reflective of Fisk. He believes that there is a uniqueness to an institution and
that its program should reflect this. A student de-
sirous of enrolling at Fisk on the undergraduate level
should go there knowing what Fisk emphasizes. These
are the kinds of expectations that we would like students to have, argues Smith. The same principle is
applicable at the graduate level. This particular
stance is reflected adequately in this seminar. There
is a whole gap of concern, omissions and commissions
about the Black aged. This seminar has sought to address itself to these issues and problems. In the same
way, the curriculum in "Social Gerontology" at Fisk
should certainly reflect that particular concern, concludes the writer.

15.   BLACK AGED AND BLACK ORGANIZATIONS

Coiro, Cynthia. "Why The National Caucus On Black Aged?"
Harvest Year, Vol. 11, November, 1971, pp. 13-18.

The writer argues that there is a definite need for
The National Caucus On Black Aged because The Black
Aged have special problems and concerns that are different than those of the White elderly. This organization is the official spokesman for the Black Aged
and espouses their causes at the local, state, and
national levels. The author gives an excellent argument for such an organization.

Jackson, Hobart C.   "National Caucus On The Black Aged: A
     Progress Report." Aging and Human Development, Vol.2,
     August, 1971, pp. 226-231.

     The Chairman of the National Caucus on The Black Aged
     (NCBA) discusses the "Formation of NCBA," "NCBA Acti-
     vities," and "The Work Ahead." He points out that
     with the cooperation of the U.S. Senate Special Com-
     mittee on Aging, and Dr. Inable Lindsay, the NCBA has
     been able to update certain information on the Black
     Elderly with respect to their life style, geographical
     distribution, estimated average income and assets, in-
     cidence and extent of chronic illness, longevity ex-
     pectations, employment patterns, quality of housing,
     effectiveness of Federal programs, and in a few other
     areas. Jackson concludes that one of the great bar-
     riers to the accomplishment of the NCBA, however, is
     the absence of current definitive usable data.

Jackson, Jacquelyne J.   "The National Center on Black
     Aged: A Challenge To Gerontologists." Gerontologist,
     Vol. 14, June, 1974, pp. 194, 196.

     The author states that gerontologists can meet the
     challenge of the National Center on Black Aged (NCBA)
     by:
               Becoming active members of NCBA.
               Sharing all relevant materials and ideas.
               Using individuals knowledgeable about Blacks
                    in the United States as key spokesmen about
                    Blacks.
               Encouraging aged Blacks to increase, where
                    necessary, their active political involve-
                    ment on local, state, and national levels.
               Involving more Blacks at all governmental and
                    private levels in planning stages for the
                    aged.
               Encouraging and aiding Black participation in
                    undergraduate, graduate, and other train-
                    ing programs from recruitment through
                    successful program completion.
               Electing political officials and legislators
                    who shall reduce racism and make certain
                    that old Blacks shall not live in poverty
                    and substandard housing.
               Recognizing that Blacks constitute a legitimate
                    and separate minority group within the
                    United States.
               Reducing efforts to lump Blacks as a minority
                    group with other legitimate minority groups,
                    such as Native Americans, and such illegiti-
                    mate minority groups as the aged, homo-
                    sexuals, and fat people.
               Helping to make real the major recommendations
                    made by the Special Concerns Session on

(Jackson, Jacquelyne J.)

        Aging and Aged Blacks at the 1971 White
House Conference on Aging, including NCBA's
"Social Security Proposal" to reduce
existing racial inequities in the distribution of OASDHI income to primary beneficiaries.
Urging the most appropriate and feasible
collection, presentation, and interpretation
of data about aging and aged Blacks by the
federal government.
Encouraging others to know and understand
realistically various patterns and processes of aging among Blacks.
Helping to increase the life expectancies and
longevities of Black males and females.

Kastenbaum, Robert J. "National Caucus on The Black Aged
(Editorial)." Aging and Human Development, Vol. 2,
1971, pp. 1-2.

The editor of the above journal points out that to be
Black and aged is truly to be in double jeopardy. He
also declares that there is a huge gap in our knowledge and understanding of Black aging. Prof. Kastenbaum concludes that the National Caucus on the Black
Aged is trying to inform the public about the special
problems of the Black aged. He also states that we
cannot claim to have developed a comprehensive science
of human aging when we know next to nothing about
those Black Americans who grow old--and those who do
not.

16. BLACK AGED AND VOLUNTEER SERVICES

Faulkner, Audrey Olsen. "The Black Aged As Good Neighbors:
An Experiment in Volunteer Service." Gerontologist,
Vol. 15, December, 1975, pp. 554-559.

The author asserts that there should be more testing
of the central hypothesis that self-image can be en-
hanced in the Black elderly by voluntary service to
others. If proof is forthcoming that the volunteer
program does indeed enrich the life of the Black senior, we will need to reach out for volunteers as we
now attempt to reach out to the potential recipients
of direct social services. Social workers can then
be less concerned about what the volunteer produces
for others and accept as most valuable the positive
results of volunteering. The writer concludes that
careful attention must be given to the tasks projected
for the volunteers. These should clearly provide special enrichment to the elderly Black population but
should not be the basic services that are provided to

(Faulkner, Audrey Olsen)

other populations by paid personnel, such as homemak-
ers, home health aides, information and referral service, nutrition services, etc.

17.   BLACK AGED AND LEGAL SERVICES

Grilfix, Michael. "Minority Elders: Legal Problems and
    the Need for Legal Services." Comprehensive Service
    Delivery System for The Minority Aged. E. Percil
    Stanford, Editor. San Diego, Calif. Center on Aging,
    School of Social Work, San Diego State University,
    1977, pp. 131-141.

The writer points out that particular legal problems
of elder minority persons include the following: (1)
They suffer from an extraordinarily high incidence of
poverty. (2) They are more dependent on public benefits and encounter more difficulties in obtaining
them. (3) They may be more susceptible to consumer
fraud and consumer abuses than Anglo elders. (4)
They are beset by problems that may be unique to their
race. (5) They suffer from the residual effects of
discrimination--both individual and institutional--
experiences at younger ages. Although some steps
have been taken to address these problems, our legal
institutions have not satisfied them. Nor, for that
matter, have legal service programs for elders been
sufficiently sensitive to minority persons, argues
the author. By identifying a number of the most
salient issues and suggesting remedial measures, it
is the hope of the author that more attention will be
given minority elders by legal service providers.
It is also the express hope of the author to involve
more minority legal workers in redressing problem
areas too long ignored.

18.   BLACK AGED AND LEISURE TIME

Anderson, Monroe. "The Pains and Pleasure of Black Folks,"
    Ebony, March, 1973, pp. 123-130.

The author points out that in 1973 about 60 percent
of the Black aged still lives in the South and the
greatest single concentration of them can be found
in New York City. It is also mentioned that 20 percent of the Black aged have no living children and
that the majority of those with children do not live
with them. Many Black aged feel that besides poverty, the major psychological problems of being old are
that many times you are lonely, you do not have many
friends left and you do not have anything to do.
Several Black aged women are interviewed in this article and they tell what it is like to be old, female,
poor, and Black.

Lambing, Mary L. Brooks. "Social Class Living Patterns of
Retired Negroes." Gerontologist, Vol. 12, Autumn,
Part 1, 1972, pp. 285-289.

This study investigates the life-style of American
Blacks retiring from the minor professions, from
stable blue-collar work, and from the service occupations, domestic work, and common labor. Data were collected through interviews with 33 men and 68 women
ranging in age from 48 to 105. Income differentials
and leisure-time activities were found to have implications for planners in recreation and social welfare.
Dr. Lambing believes future studies of the Black aged
might focus on two groups not included here, those
retiring from the major professions, such as law and
medicine, and those who need the help of Public Assistance payments but are not willing to have a lien
on their property in order to qualify. She concludes
that many older Blacks in the lower classes have inadequate income even though they may have pensions or
Old Age Assistance; those without the additional help
of Social Security benefits must live a spartan life
indeed. Social planners need to recognize these
shortcomings in the present system. Gerontologists
planning recreational facilities for Blacks can benefit by recognizing social class differences in leisure-time activities, argues the author.

Marshall, Marion. "Differential Use of Time." Workshop
on Community Services and The Black Elderly. Richard
H. Davis, Editor. Los Angeles: Andrus Gerontology
Center, University of Southern California, 1972, pp.
12-16.

The author feels that it is much more difficult to get
the older Black person to use his leisure time in involvement activities, for they have not had this encouragement from society. Marshall concludes that
we must help the Black elderly to move away from being
told what to do. They must plan together what to do
and then take the responsibility of getting it done.

19. BLACK AGED AND EDUCATION

"College Coed--At 76." Ebony, December, 1966, pp. 79-83.

This article discusses Mrs. Caroline Cooper who attended Fresno City College. The learning process, as
Mrs. Cooper sees it, is not only desirable for the
older person, it is essential. She argues "the greatest and most tragic waste of our nation's economy is
the waste of human minds." Mrs. Cooper concludes
"that many older people's minds die long before their
bodies do. There's nothing left for them but their
bodily bulk. Then they just sit around and gossip.

("College Coed--At 76,")

Gossip becomes a disease with them, a disease that eventually eats away their remaining time. It's a horrible waste of human life, and I refuse to be among the waste," declared Mrs. Cooper.

Ford, Johnny. "Black Aged in The Future in a Predominantly Black Southern Town." Proceedings of Black Aged in The Future. Jacquelyne J. Jackson, Editor. Durham, N. C.: Center for The Study of Aging and Human Development, Duke University, 1973, pp. 1-10.

The author discusses Tuskegee, Alabama as a site for a comprehensive Housing complex for the elderly. Such a complex would provide social services, as well as housing, recreation, health services, economic opportunities, and social activities. He declares that those who are concerned about the aged in this country should look South, and to create strategies which will develop and mold the resources for the aged ending up in the South. Ford concludes that Black and poor people, and older people especially, need money and resources, not words.

Jackson, Jacquelyne J. "Aged Negroes: Their Cultural Departures From Statistical Stereotypes and Rural-Urban Differences." Gerontologist, Vol. 10, Summer, 1970, pp. 140-145.

The major purpose of this article is that of suggesting some areas where aged Blacks tend to become "cultural departurers" from statistical stereotypes and also of suggesting certain variables which may be useful in distinguishing between rural and urban aged Blacks. Essentially, both tasks were only partially successful, due to the scarcity of available data about aged Blacks and, no doubt, to the value judgments imposed upon those data. Given those limitations, however, Black aged tend to depart from such statistical stereotypes as those which hold that their marital statuses are significantly different from those of White aged; that their life expectancies are typically less than those of Whites (they may be longer at the later age periods); that they differ significantly from Whites by importance placed upon their families, or that they are more religious, in poorer health, or less active in formal organizations than Whites, concludes Dr. Jackson.

_____. "A Bicentennial Tribute To Older Blacks: Black Professionals in North Carolina." Black Aging, Vol. 2, Nos. 2 and 3, December, 1976 and February, 1977, pp. 9-21.

This essay, which concentrates upon the relative

(Jackson, Jacquelyne J.)

growth, individual contributions, and opportunities
for professional education for Blacks in North Carolina, showed a numerical increase in Black professionals between 1930 and 1970, but no real growth or
progress within their professional status. In comparison with all professionally employed persons within
the state, Blacks were better off in 1930 than in
1970. Non-Black professional employment was much more
swift in growth over that time. The unfortunate
trend of decreased Black employment within the labor
force was quite alarming. The vignettes about four
Black professionals born between 1763 and 1923 (John
Chavis, Joseph Charles Price, Charlotte Hawkins Brown,
and Reginald Armistice Hawkins) provides contrasting
examples of Black professional contributions to the
state's well being. The abbreviated review of state
provisions for Black professional education since the
American Revolution showed better opportunities now
than ever before, with those opportunities having
been expanded primarily through Black and federal
pressures, and with the state usually restricting itself to minimal federal or accrediting requirements,
concludes the author.

Smith, Stanley H. "The Older Rural Negro." Older Rural
Americans: A Sociological Perspective. E. Grant
Youmans, Editor. Lexington: University of Kentucky
Press, 1967, pp. 262-80.

This article discusses some selected demographic characteristics of aged rural Blacks; data on educational
level, employment, and income. In all cases, aged
rural Blacks are far behind in all these categories.
The writer also gives some data on the involvement of
aged rural Blacks in American life; and a small a-
mount of data which are designed to give an assessment
of some of the subjective reactions of aged rural
Blacks to their social and economic conditions. The
author concludes that aged rural Blacks have three
things against them: old age, rural residence, and
minority-group status.

Tucker, Charles J. "Changes in Age Composition of The
Rural Black Population of the South From 1950-1970."
Phylon, Vol. 33, Fall, 1974, pp. 268-275.

The writer states that of a decline of 1.5 million
persons in the South's rural Black population between
1950 and 1970, a net minimum of 1.9 million Blacks
moved to cities within the region or moved outside the
region altogether, therefore, accounting for all the
decrease. Had it not been for relatively high fer-
tility among those who remained, declines would have

(Tucker, Charles J.)

been greater still. The estimates of migration presented in this paper are based on the application of
1950-1970 cohort ratios for the total U.S. Black population during the period and do not include estimates of migration among those persons born after
1950. These ratios were applied to the age structure
of the Black rural population of the South in 1950.
He said for total losses, the heaviest were obviously
found among the farm segment of the rural population.
The farm population declined by no less than 86 percent over the twenty years. Within this population,
losses were heaviest among farm youth who were younger
than 20 years of age in 1950, most of whom must have
migrated to urban places. For older persons who had
already become established in farm occupations by
1950, migration was not as heavy and when it occurred,
was probably directed to nonfarm areas or entailed a
shift in occupation from farm to other activities
without a movement to urban places and jobs. The writer concludes that shifts in occupation or residence
on the part of many farm Blacks of older ages had the
effect of increasing the number of nonfarm Blacks by
more than 50 percent over the twenty year period.
Young adult age groups barely increased in number at
all. There is little wonder, then, that the dependency ratio of nonfarm Blacks increased drastically
due to the shortage of young adults, contends Tucker.

20. BLACK AGED AND LONELINESS

Kivett, Vira R. "Loneliness and The Rural Black Elderly:
    Perspectives on Intervention." Black Aging, Vol. 3,
    Nos. 4 and 5, April and June, 1978, pp. 160-166.

Results from this article show that three out of five
older rural Blacks surveyed experienced varying bouts
of loneliness which could be partially explained by
intra-group differences on several population characteristics. Social rather than physical factors
generally contributed to loneliness by creating the
social as well as emotional isolation of older adults.
Inadequate transportation and the loss of a spouse
through death, separation or divorce were significant
influences on both occasional and frequent loneliness.
The flexibility to travel from one place to another,
whether it be for the purpose of shopping, visiting
with family, or for other reasons seemed to be crucial
to feelings of loneliness, states the author. The
frequency with which older rural Blacks telephoned
friends, relatives, or others appeared to be an index
to the extent of loneliness being incurred. The frequently lonely showed considerable effort to circum-
vent their feelings of loneliness through a "reaching

(Kivett, Vira R.)

out" to others via the telephone. Despite the observation of the similarity between the occasionally and
the frequently lonely, important distinctions could
be made between the two groups based on adequacy of
eyesight, marital status, and educational level. The
observation that older Blacks who were frequently
rather than sometimes lonely were more likely to have
poor eyesight, to have a higher education, to be married rather than divorced, and to report that they had
no one in whom they could trust or confide suggested
the relatively weak role that marriage may play as an
emotional support among certain groups of older married Black adults, specifically, the higher educated,
visually impaired, argues the writer. Several variables failed to separate older Blacks according to frequency of loneliness. Some appeared to be suppressed
because of the relative homogeneity of the rural sample, i.e., socioeconomic characteristics based on previous work type and education. The suppressed variables in question included adequacy of income, and
self-rated health. An earlier analysis of data that
contained both White and Black subgroups showed self-
rated health significantly differentiated older adults
according to loneliness, concludes the author.

21. BLACK AGED AND SUICIDE

Hill, Robert. "A Profile of Black Aged." Proceedings of
The Research Conference on Minority Group Aged in
the South. Jacquelyne J. Jackson, Editor. Durham,
N. C.: Center for the Study of Aging and Human Development, Duke University Medical Center, 1972, pp. 92-
96.

The writer states that because of the historic oppression of Blacks one would ordinarily predict that
suicide rates would be greater for Blacks than Whites.
It is also interesting to note that the gap is even
greater among the elderly. For example, Black males,
65-69, have a suicide rate of 12.8, but 65-69 year-old
White males have a suicide rate of 35.6. And when
we look at those between 75 and 79, the suicide rate
for Black men is 15.0, but it is 42.5 among elderly
White men, contends Dr. Hill. One of the most interesting aspects of the suicide rates is that they are
lowest among Black women, who are probably the most
oppressed group in America, according to Dr. Hill.
Thus, the story of the Black elderly is really an in-
spiring saga of courage and determination against ad-
versity. In many ways, the elderly Blacks, perhaps
more than any other age group, best exemplify the historic fortitude and resilience of Black people in America, concludes the author.

Swanson, William C. and Carl L. Harter. "How Do Elderly
    Blacks Cope in New Orleans." <u>Aging and Human Devel-</u>
    <u>opment</u>, Vol. 2, August, 1971, pp. 210-216.

This article was based on case histories from a representative sample of twenty Black men and women age
fifty-five or older residing in New Orleans. The authors provide several insights into significant life
features of elderly Blacks in that city. First, it
was found that many of these Blacks suffered from financial and health problems; yet, by no means did
they feel that life was unbearable. Secondly, these
elderly Blacks do not feel they have ever had any
serious personal problems. Thirdly, these poor elderly Blacks are <u>NOT</u> high suicide risks. The authors
conclude that though they may be poor, old, sick, and
Black, being alive is still good and precious--to the
aged Blacks in New Orleans.

22. BLACK AGED AND POLITICS

Jackson, Jacquelyne J. "NCBA, Black Aged and Politics."
    <u>Annuals of The American Academy of Political and</u>
    <u>Social Science</u>, Vol. 415, 1974, pp. 138-159.

The author discusses the National Caucus on Black Aged
and the needs for such an organization. She argues
that it will only be an effective agency for dealing
with the problems of the Black aged if it has the
necessary support from both Blacks and Whites. Dr.
Jackson surmises that this organization, like others,
should be free from politics. Unfortunately, it is
not, she concludes.

Robinson, Henry. "Political Action and The Black Aged."
    <u>Action For Aged Blacks: When?: A Conference of The</u>
    <u>National Caucus on The Black Aged</u>. Jacquelyne J.
    Jackson, Editor. Washington, D. C.: National Caucus
    on The Black Aged, 1973, pp. 32-34.

The author states that in 1970 there were nearly
1,500,000 Blacks 65 years or older making up about 8%
of the Black population. He argues that if this large
proportion of people were brought together as a co-
hesive force they could play a significant role in the
political area. Robinson argues that the Black aged
have all the problems of the aged plus the handicaps
of discrimination, poverty, poor housing, inferior
health facilities, and faulty nutrition, to name just
a few. The writer asserts that the Black aged must
not only register to vote, he must exercise that vote
on election day.

23. MYTHS ABOUT THE BLACK AGED

Jackson, Jacquelyne J. "Black Aged in Quest of the Phoe-
    nix." Triple Jeopardy--Myth or Reality. Washington,
    D. C.: National Council on the Aged, 1972.

The author, while not denying the heterogeneity among
Black elderly, forcefully argues that "race is a reality and we should not deny it . . . . Insofar as
Black old people are concerned, I think that we
should not now begin to treat them as if they were the
same as White old people. They are not." Racism has
adversely affected their preparation for old age, concludes Dr. Jackson.

_____ and Bertram E. Walls. "Myths and Realities
About Aged Blacks." Readings in Gerontology. Mollie
Brown, Editor. St. Louis, Mo.: C. V. Mosby Co.,
1978, pp. 95-113.

The development of gerontological knowledge about
Blacks has been hampered severely by racial biases
and vested interests. The significant differences between aged Blacks and Whites typically stressed by advocates for aged Blacks are largely myths. Gerontologists have generally abetted the perpetuation of
these myths through ineffectual controls of the variable of race in their contrasts of aged Blacks and
Whites. This study, which was primarily concerned
with the resolution of prevalent myths about aged
Blacks and Whites, was based on an analysis of the
1974 Harris data about aging attitudes and behaviors
in the United States. The finding of a general absence of any significant racial differences between
paired groups of low- and high-income aged and young
Blacks and Whites in the Harris survey suggested
strongly the vast similarity of aging process and
patterns among American Blacks and Whites, argue the
writers. An examination of variables related to so-
ciodemographic characteristics, aging images and attitudes, aging activities, aging problems, and patterns of familial assistance showed striking similarities between low-income, as well as high-income, aged
Blacks and Whites. For example, comparisons of appropriately controlled groups of aged Blacks and
Whites by income levels indicated insignificant differences by such variables as activities, instrumental
assistance from and to families, religion, and health.
The few significant differences reported herein would
undoubtedly wash out with more stringent controls for
socioeconomic status. In other words, current myths
about significant differences between aged Blacks and
Whites have little, if any, validity, state the writers. The authors conclude that the most important
implication of their study for aging programs involv-

(Jackson, Jacquelyne J. and Bertram E. Walls)

ing Blacks is the need to structure such programs on
adequate knowledge about the conditions under which
race is and is not a factor. Furthermore, advocates
for racially separated programs should avoid hiding
behind aged Blacks when they are clearly more concerned about building Black power bases for themselves. Finally, aging training programs should
place greater emphasis on training individuals of
various races to provide services to individuals of
various races. They should also aid their students in
distinguishing clearly between significant differences
between populations, such as aged Blacks and Whites,
and significant differences between individuals who
happen to be aged Blacks or Whites, surmise the authors.

24. BLACK AGED AND SEX

West, Malcolm R. "Who Says You Get Too Old To Enjoy Sex?
Not These Youngsters!" Jet, August 11, 1977, pp. 22-
24.

This article discusses the sex lives of several of
Chicago's senior citizens who have been experiencing
the joys of sex for more than sixty years. These aged
Blacks discuss how frequently they have sex. Some
stated they had sex every week. Others declared they
had sex every other week and still others said once a
month.

25. BLACK AGED AND THE FEDERAL GOVERNMENT

Flemming, Arthur C. "Action and Aged Blacks: The Post-
White House Conference on Aging." Action For Aged
Blacks: When? A Conference of The National Caucus on
The Black Aged. Jacquelyne J. Jackson, Editor. Wash-
ington, D. C.: National Caucus on The Aged, 1973,
pp. 43-51.

The writer discusses his nomination as Commissioner on
Aging and what he would do, that would affect Black
people, in that position. He stated that he wanted
Blacks in policy making positions in his organization
and on all policy making levels of government, especially those that affect the aged, including the Social
and Rehabilitation Service, Social Security Administration, U.S. Department of Agriculture, Department of
Health, Education and Welfare and the Office of Economic Opportunity.

Jackson, Jacquelyne J. "Aged Blacks: A Potpourri in The
Direction of The Reduction of Inequities." Phylon,
Vol. 32, Fall, 1971, pp. 260-280.

(Jackson, Jacquelyne J.)

The triple focus of this article is upon (a) a description and analysis of Southern urban Black grandparental roles, emphasizing certain implications for
current policies surrounding Black aged; (b) the
National Caucus on the Black Aged, stressing its ur-
gent missions of dramatizing the plight of the Black
aged and having a significant impact upon the forthcoming 1971 White House Conference on Aging, where
policy recommendations for the aged in the decade
ahead will be formulated, as well as its general concern for increasing substantially services to, training for, and research about Black aged; and (c) a
specific proposal to reduce the minimum age-eligibility requirements for recipients of Old-Age, Survivors,
Disability and Health Insurance (OASDHI, a form of
Social Security) so as to reduce the racial inequities now extant, wherein Blacks are far less likely to
receive proportionate benefits as Whites, even though
they may be very likely to have invested proportion-
ately more of their life-time earnings into Social
Security, inasmuch as they tend to die earlier than
do Whites. Dr. Jackson argues that the interfacing of
these foci occurred largely in that the grandparental
data point toward the need for improved economic and
housing conditions for grandparents, for their children and for their children's children. The National
Caucus on the Black Aged is significantly concerned
about improving these adverse conditions and, in this
connection, seeks assistance from all relevant resources (including those Blacks who are not yet aged).
The writer concludes that the specific proposal to
realize greater racial equity between aged Whites and
Blacks is one response to the need to improve the de-
plorable income plight of many Black aged: in this
case, a specific improvement in obtaining benefits
which Black aged themselves have earned.

Mitchell, Parren J. "Mutual National Caucus on The Black
    Aged (NCBA) and The Congressional Black Caucus (CBC)
    Concerns About Aged Blacks and Recommended Legislation
    For Action." Action For Aged Blacks: When? A Con-
    ference of The National Caucus on The Black Aged.
    Jacquelyne J. Jackson, Editor. Washington, D. C.:
    National Caucus on The Black Aged, 1973, pp. 76-87.

This Black Congressman from Maryland states what the
CBC was doing to help the Black aged. He declares
that the astronomically high unemployment among Black
people has significant implications for senior Black
citizens; because if Blacks are unemployed at a high
rate, then they can not possibly help support Black
senior citizens. The Congressman also pointed out
that the CBC was working with the NCBA in the develop-

(Mitchell, Parren J.)

ment of a legislative program that would implement
some of the recommendations made at the 1971 White
House Conference on Aging.

Sheppard, N. Alan. "A Federal Perspective on The Black
     Aged: From Concern To Action." Aging, September-
     October, 1978, pp. 28-32.

This article highlights the need for Federal efforts
in the aging field by presenting a profile of the elderly population and their concerns/needs. He contends that the Federal Government needs to provide a
perspective on the minority aged, in general, and
aged Blacks in particular; to show by example how a
Federal agency such as the Federal Council on the Aging can move from concern to action for the minority
aged. Dr. Sheppard concludes that the commitment of
the Federal government must be firm, steadfast, and
built upon a sound and effective strategy for dealing
with the Black Aged.

26. MINORITY AGED

Lipman, Aaron. "Ethnic and Minority Group Content For
     Courses in Aging." Gerontology In Higher Education:
     Perspectives and Issues, Papers From The 1977 Meeting
     of The Association For Gerontology in Higher Education.
     Mildren M. Seltzer, et al., Editors. Belmont, Calif.:
     Wadsworth Publishing Co., Inc., 1978, pp. 223-227.

The author points out that while we have become aware
that within that numerical minority there is a subgroup of racial and ethnic minority aged population
clusters that must be clearly delineated, effectively
researched, and the results disseminated in texts and
lectures that teach social gerontology. The four major minority groups that have been distinguished in
the United States and which should be included in the
initial thrust, are the American Indian or native Americans, Black Americans, Asian Americans and Spanish-
speaking Americans. In studying the minority aged,
contends the author, we need to collect a body of
knowledge which will indicate uniformities in the
minority experience of aging, as contrasted with the
dominant group, as well as showing the effects of subcultural differences between various minorities. The
author continues to argue that the fund of knowledge
we already possess concerning the minority elderly indicates that as a group, they are more economically
disadvantaged than those elderly that belong to the
dominant group. Yet while attention has been given to
social class differences research has neglected to
account for variations within or across class lines

(Lipman, Aaron)

due to the interplay of racial or ethnic factors.
Part of the problem with data concerning the poor is
the confounding of the concepts "poor" and "minority."
For the total population at all ages the likelihood of
being poor if one is a member of a minority is four
times as great as for that of the dominant group,
states the author. By the time a person reaches old
age, that proportion is down to twice as great. This
is not necessarily due to an improvement in the fortunes of the poor elderly minority member as he gets
old, but more probably to the fact that so small a
number survive to old age. In 1975, the median income
for White families was $14,268, compared with $9,551
for Hispanics and $8,779 for Black families. "Nearly
27 percent of Hispanics were below the federally defined poverty level of $5,500 for an urban family of
four, compared with 9.7 percent of Whites and 31.3
percent of Blacks," concludes the writer. In 1975,
for those 65 years and over, 13.4 percent of the
Whites were below the poverty level compared with 32.7
percent of the Hispanics and 36.3 percent of the
Blacks. The writer also concludes that it is important to include material about minority groups in our
curricula on aging for a number of reasons: There is
the purely epistemological aim of scientifically ex-
panding our theoretical generalizable base of knowledge concerning the total gerontic population. Secondly, comparative studies on the adjustment of different groups to aging could identify the dynamics
that contribute to that adjustment and by identifying
those coping structures and mechanisms which work for
variant subcultural groups in our society, we might
also refine our knowledge of the dominant group adaptation process. Finally, knowledge about minority
groups would help generate action programs and policies targeted for those individuals who, as a consequence of their membership in an ethnic or racial minority subgroup, have not been reached by programs
which were designed by and for the dominant White,
contends the author.

Moss, Frank E. and Val J. Halamandaris.   "No Vacancy for
    Minority Groups: Aged Blacks." Too Old, Too Sick,
    Too Bad: Nursing Homes in America. Germantown, Mary-
    land: Aspen Systems Corp., 1977, pp. 117-121.

The writers state that older Blacks are twice as likely to be poor; 50 percent live in poverty as compared
with 23 percent for Whites. While over half of them
continue to live in the South, the migration of this
minority group into urban areas has created over-
crowded conditions, poor health, drug addiction, and
social and personal violence. To the Black American

(Moss, Frank E. and Val J. Halamandaris)

this means a higher mortality rate at every stage of
life. From 45 to 64, Black women have twice the mortality rate of White women; from 55 to 64, the mortality for Black men is ten percent higher than for
White men. Despite higher incidences of acute and
chronic disease, an elderly Black sees a physician at
an average annual rate of 4.9 visits as compared with
a White's 6.1 visits. Aged Blacks are experiencing
no temporary aberration, but rather the continuing
effect of poverty and racism. "Now in their golden
years, they have relinquished whatever hopes they had
--resigned to an ignominious death in a subtle form
of euthanasia," argue the authors. They declare that
since half of the 1.7 million elderly Blacks are poor,
it appears safe to assume that cost would not be an
important factor, the assumption being that the poor
are eligible for Medicaid, which now pays more than
50 percent of the nation's home bill, according to
the authors. While there are obvious social and cultural differences between Blacks and the White majority population, these differences rank well behind
cost and discrimination as a reason for Blacks' not
entering nursing homes. Like Asians, they continue to
have a reputation for "taking care of their own." Representatives of the Black community noted that this
tradition continues for the principal reason that
there is no place beyond the bosom of the family that
an elderly Black can find supportive services, conclude the writers.

27. COMPARATIVE BLACK AND WHITE AGED

Clemente, Frank, et al. "The Participation of Black Aged
    in Voluntary Associations." Journal of Gerontology,
    Vol. 30, July, 1975, pp. 469-478.

Racial differences in membership in and attendance of
voluntary associations were analyzed for comparable
samples of 753 Black and 260 White residents of Philadelphia age 65 and over. A hypothesis suggesting
aged Blacks have higher rates of participation than
aged Whites was derived from the literature and tested
by regression analysis. The authors declare potenti-
ally confounding variables, e.g., health and socioeconomic status, were entered into the regression
equation as controls. They state the results of the
regression analysis indicated the Black aged belonged
to more associations than the White aged and had higher rates of attendance. The writers conclude examination of findings previously reported indicate part
of the difference is due to the greater participation
of aged Blacks in church-related groups. Implications of the findings are briefly discussed.

Creecy, Robert F. and Roosevelt Wright. "Morale and In-
    formal Activity With Friends Among Black and White
    Elderly." Gerontologist, Vol. 19, No. 6, December,
    1979, pp. 544-547.

This article examines the nature of the relationship
between informal activity with friends and morale
among a sample of White and Black elderly. The data
indicate a statistically significant relationship between these variables within the White sub-sample, but
within the Black sub-sample this relationship was substantially insignificant. The major implication of
this research revolves around the finding that informal activity with friends was not associated with
morale among Black elderly. While it was suggested
that the lack of intimacy in the friendships of Blacks
may account for this finding, this was not tested
since a measure of intimacy was not included in the
data, according to the writers. The writers conclude
that the future efforts of policy-makers and planners
and the activities of practitioners should focus on
the development and implementation of improved social
service programs that enhance the opportunity for
social interactions and friendship formation among the
Black elderly, thereby minimizing the risk of social
isolation among this population subgroup.

Durant, Thomas J., Jr. "Residence, Race and Sex Differ-
    ences in Level of Alienation Among the Aged." Journal
    of Social and Behavioral Sciences, Vol. 24, No. 2,
    Spring, 1978, pp. 85-101.

The author tested six hypotheses with data collected
by the personal interview technique on 458 persons of
65 years of age and over from two Louisiana parishes.
The study found that all four dimensions of alienation, group isolation, powerlessness, normlessness,
and personal isolation, existed to a substantial degree
among the aged studied, but powerlessness was particularly more prevalent. Level of alienation did not
vary by rural and urban residence and in only one instance by sex. More powerlessness was found among
males than among females, and Blacks were more alien-
ated than Whites, especially in terms of group isolation. The status resource variables, especially education, were found to be greater sources of variance
in alienation than were the social interaction variables. Status resource variables also served as
greater sources of variance in alienation for Whites
than for Blacks and for urban residents over rural residents. No difference was found by sex, in this regard, according to the author.

Golden, Herbert. "Black Ageism." Social Policy, Vol. 7,
    No. 3, November/December, 1976, pp. 40-42.

The author argues that what is clear is that attempts
to apply research findings based on undifferentiated
comparisons between Black and White elderly toward the
solution of problems faced by Black elderly are doomed
to ineffectiveness. Social scientists by and large
agree that race is an American social reality and as
such must be regarded as an independent variable in
any study attempting to offer policy and/or planning
objectives. It is then only when Blacks are studied
as a group without necessarily making comparisons to
the larger White elderly population that we will have
a good base for attacking the unique problems that
this minority group membership imposes on people's adaptation to aging, concludes the author.

Goldstein, Sidney. "Negro-White Differentials in Consumer
    Patterns of The Aged, 1960-1961." Gerontologist,
    Vol. 11, Autumn, 1971, pp. 242-249.

The writer asserts that since 1960-1961, the income
of both White and Black aged units has improved, but
even in 1968, older Black income levels were only a-
bout two-thirds as high as those of White units, and
the percentage of Black units classified as below the
poverty level remained substantial, especially for unrelated individuals. This being so, it seems likely
that important differences also continue to characterize the expenditure dimensions of the consumer behavior of White and Black aged units. The author concludes the compounding influences of age and race make
the economic situation of older Black units particularly bleak and warrants special attention to this
segment of the aged population.

Hicks, Nancy. "Life After 65." Black Enterprise, May,
    1977, pp. 18-22.

The writer points out that less than five percent of
all people over 65 live in nursing homes. About 60
percent of the Black Aged and 55 percent of the White
live in and around cities, although more than half the
Blacks are still in the South. According to Miss
Hicks about one-quarter live on farms. It is stated
that there are many reasons why a larger percentage of
Black elderly live with their children: the importance of the role of grandmother, because mother works
or is away; the need for sharing of income within a
family, including the older person's Social Security
and public assistance payments; and the respect and
sense of responsibility said to exist more strongly in
Black households, in caring for and protecting one's
parents, particularly the aged mother.

Hirsch, Carl. "A Review of Findings on Social and Economic
  Conditions of Low-Income Black and White Aged of Phil-
  adelphia." Proceedings of The Research Conference on
  Minority Group Aged in the South. Jacquelyne J. Jack-
  son, Editor. Durham, N. C.: Center for the Study of
  Aging and Human Development, Duke University Medical
  Center, 1972, pp. 63-81.

  This is a report on an inquiry into the conditions of
  urban low-income elderly persons. The study population of this research was selected to yield information about both low-income aged Blacks and Whites.
  Virtually all of the more than 1,000 persons interviewed may be classified as low-income. About 3/4 of
  those interviewed were Black. The consideration
  prompting the study was a need to explore the role of
  the resources and agencies available to the aged and
  the conditions and adjustments of the aged. The deci-
  sion to focus upon the low-income elderly was prompted
  by a number of considerations. Among them was the
  finding that most earlier studies of the aged had utilized samples from either of two groups: institutionalized aged or middle-class aged. The need is great
  for comparable data on the aged living within the community, but in poor economic circumstances, concludes
  the author.

Hirsch, Carl. "Serving Aged Residents of Central City
  Neighborhoods." Challenges Facing Senior Centers in
  the Nineteen Seventies. Alice G. Wolfson, Editor.
  New York: National Council On The Aging, 1968, pp.
  134-145.

  This article discusses aged Blacks in Philadelphia.
  The author found evidence of a higher rate of affili-
  ation with voluntary associations among low-income
  Blacks than among low-income Whites. The difference
  in the writer's sample is perhaps explained by the
  greater rate of religious activity among Black respondents and their greater potential for memberships in
  church or religious groups. The essential conclusions,
  drawn from Dr. Hirsch's study, relates to serving that
  particular minority of aged persons who reside in the
  low socio-economic neighborhoods of central cities,
  concern: the lack of effective communication between
  agencies and the aged; the demonstrated potential of
  an outreach mechanism that attempts to deliver coor-
  dinated services to the aged individual at his door;
  and the importance of the aged person's concept of
  life space and the functional relevance of services to
  him which, if ignored by those delivering and developing services, can hinder and retard utilization, concludes the author.

Hirsch, Carl, et al. "Homogeneity and Heterogeneity Among
    Low-Income Negro and White Aged." Research Planning
    and Action for The Elderly: The Power and Potential
    of Social Science. Donald P. Kent, et al., Editors.
    New York: Behavioral Publications, Inc., 1972, pp.
    484-500.

The availability of medical care to low-income aged
in a metropolitan setting is well documented by the
data from this study. More than one-third of the
study group (again, no racial differences) had had an
eye examination during the previous year. More than
80% wore glasses. While only a fifth had visited a
dentist during the preceeding year, 60% had dentures.
Again, difference between the races was slight. These
data give too favorable a picture. A contextual analysis and the case material collected bring to light
less favorable aspects. Clinics and hospitals often
are located too far from the neighborhoods of the low-
income aged. Public transportation is frequently non-
existent, often inconvenient, and almost always too
expensive. Health personnel at times fail to commun-
icate with the old. At times the health professional
assumes a greater medical sophistication on the part
of the aged patient than exists; and at other times
the health workers are amazingly blind to the social
needs of the elderly patient, declare the authors.
His medical needs will be well diagnosed and the appropriate prophylactic prescribed; but at the same
time his social needs will be completely disregarded
with the result that the latter quite negate the
hoped-for medical therapy. Since, in many respects,
the Black church follows a traditional pattern, it may
more nearly meet the cultural expectations of the present group of elderly. Conceivably, the greater interest of the Black aged in religion reflects not a
greater inner need but rather a greater adaptability
of the Black church to the desires of the aged. The
writers argue that perhaps the White church in its
open efforts to reach the young has developed a service and message less congenial to the White aged.
The authors examined differences by race and sex and
found both heterogeneity and homogeneity between and
among members of both racial groups. Age has only
been introduced into discussion occasionally although
they have some indication that the importance of age
varies by race-sex group according to the charac ter-
istic being considered. Further analysis of age differences among the aged group is certainly planned,
conclude the writers.

Hudson, Gossie Harold. "The Black Aged: Some Reflections
    By A Layman." Proceedings Of the Workshop Series On
    The Black Aging and Aged and The Conference On The
    Black Aged and Aging. Jean Dorsett-Robinson, et al.,
    Editors. Carbondale, Ill.: College of Human Re-
    sources, Southern Illinois University, 1974, pp. 113-
    119.

The author contends that the social and economic problems of older Blacks, compounded by race and age, are
particularly bleak and warrant special attention in
the literature. Contemporary scholars in the field of
gerontology generally agree that the difficulties of
unemployment are more severe among non-white workers
who are doubly disadvantaged because they are often
discriminated against on the basis of both age and
minority group status. In fact, unemployment among
elderly Blacks is almost triple the rate of that experienced by elderly Whites. However, the socio-economic problems confronting the Black aged are undoubtedly a continuation of earlier disadvantages rather
than solely a reflection of currently inadequate income. Therefore, to reduce poverty in old age, deprivation must be attacked in the early years, argues Dr.
Hudson. To be sure, adequate income cannot be abruptly established at age 65 or age 62. Dr. Hudson declares that a mere perusal of the sources will show
that despite the general upgrading of the labor force
in this generation, Blacks are still far too well
represented among those who are employed in jobs at
which even White workers average low earnings throughout a lifetime. Moreover, current efforts have not
resulted in better employment opportunities for Blacks,
states the writer. This suggests, of course, that
when younger Blacks reach old age, they will probably
share in the poverty that earlier stalked them and
their children just because of the color of their
skin, concludes the author.

_____. "Some Special Problems Of Older Black Ameri-
cans." Crisis, Vol. 83, No. 3, March, 1976, pp. 88-
90.

The writer points out that about 16 percent of all
Black households are headed by elderly persons. Among
the Black elderly, one-third of the women and one-
fourth of the men live alone. About one-fourth of all
the old men never had any children. About one-half
live in poverty, and well over one-half reside in
substandard housing. While the life expectancy of
Black males continues to be approximately seven years
less than that of either Black females or White males,
those Blacks who have survived to very old age have
a higher remaining life expectancy than do Whites.
When younger Blacks reach old age, they will probably

(Hudson, Gossie Harold)

share in the poverty that earlier stalked them and
their children because of the color of their skins
and the rampant racism in the society. Therefore, to
reduce poverty in old age, relative deprivation must
be attacked in the early years because adequate income
cannot be abruptly established at age 65, contends Dr.
Hudson. The total mean income for all aged Black
females is only 59.7 percent as much as that of their
male counterparts; those with high school and college
education measure 54.7 and 69.2 percent, respectively.
Actually the same type of ever-widening gaps in income patterns when Blacks and Whites in the United
States are compared over the past few decades are also
present when comparing Black females and males. As
the absolute income earnings of Whites are becoming
continuously larger than those of Blacks, the absolute
income earnings of Black males are also becoming continuously larger than those of Black females. In general, older Black people have had less education than
Whites and therefore have had less choice in work opportunities. The Black woman's median years of
schooling is about 6th grade, while for men it is 4th
grade. Today, about 16 percent of older Black people
are illiterate while the rate for Whites is only 2
percent. Housing, too, is poorer for aged Blacks than
for aged Whites. Less than 3 percent of the people in
nursing homes or homes for the aged are Black. Older
Blacks do not have the financial ability to enter
homes for the aged, and are often discriminated
against by the homes. In addition, few of the homes
are located in the Black community, states the writer.
An even greater problem is recognized when one knows
that most of the agencies trying to serve the Black
community are short of funds. Psychological damages
help to compound the problems of economic and social
insecurity. The development of negative self-attitudes
often causing self-hatred and rejection of others like
one's self, obsessive sensitivity, dependence, and
alienation are some of the observed consequences of
minority status. The corrosive effects of prejudice
and discrimination reach their zenith when the minority group internalizes cultural definitions of infer-
iority. "Ageism," like its cousins, "racism" and
"sexism," fosters in the older person the haunting
fear that all the stereotypes held about him are accu-
rate. The resulting passivity, anxiety, and withdrawal can be viewed as accommodative actions by the aged
as they attempt to adjust to prevailing cultural definitions. Also, the high rates of suicide, behavioral
disturbances, and mental aberrations are qualifiable
measures of the consequences of older people's encounter with institutional and personal discrimination.
Dr. Hudson concludes that these personal pathologies

(Hudson, Gossie Harold)

reflect a deep and pervasive malaise in the American social structure.

Jenkins, Mercilee M. "Age and Migration Factors in The Socioeconomic Conditions of Urban Blacks and Urban White Women." Industrial Gerontology, Vol. 9, Spring, 1971, pp. 13-17.

The writer concludes that part-time and seasonal employment or nonparticipation in the labor market are more-characteristic of Black than of White women in all three urban-size types. Among Black workers, young women in large cities enjoy the greatest occupational success, whereas older Black women in small cities usually have low-status jobs and earn the least. Extreme poverty is more frequently experienced by White families, both young and old, who have always lived in the city. For Black families, the situation is reversed; particularly in the middle-class and large urban areas it appears that migrants are not a burden to the cities as is commonly believed. As a group they are not poorly educated and prone to unemployment or welfare roles; indeed, it seems that some have actual advantages over native urbanites, concludes the author.

Kalish, Richard A. "Death and Dying: A Cross-Cultural View." Proceedings of Black Aged in The Future. Jacquelyne J. Jackson, Editor. Durham, N. C.: Center for The Study of Aging and Human Development, Duke University, 1973, pp. 11-22.

The author compares Blacks with Asians, Mexicans, and Whites in Los Angeles and concludes that Blacks displayed the greatest wish for and expectation of longer life. He argues that to understand an older person, we need to understand the general processes of aging, both social and biological; we need to recognize his particular culture, its history and its present circumstances; and we need to seek a person's strengths, while enabling him to deal more effectively with his weaknesses. Dr. Kalish points out that some of the strengths include durability, wisdom, knowledge, faith and loyalty.

Kandel, Randy F. and Marion Heider. "Friendship and Factionalism in a TRI-ETHNIC Housing Complex for The Elderly in North Miami." Anthropological Quarterly, Vol. 52, January, 1979, pp. 49-59.

The authors used conflict and environmental docility models to analyze the impact of ethnicity, architectural design and internal politics on community

(Kandel, Randy F. and Marion Heider)

formation in a U.S. Department of Housing and Development subsidized development for Black, Cuban and
White English-speaking elderly. Four interlinked
levels of community participation (dyadic friendships,
ethnic subcommunities, Tenant's Council political factionalism, and the "community-of-the-whole") are discussed with particular reference to the roles of culture brokers, the Tenant's Council's relationship to
the external political structure, and the unique psychological and social conditions of the elderly.
The authors conclude that because most residents of
communities for the elderly have nowhere else to turn,
it is a moral imperative to provide them with the largest possible range of options for achieving life satisfaction. They suggest this can best be done by de-
signing highly flexible residential arrangements and
political and social organizations in future retirement communities.

Kasschau, Patricia L. "Age and Race Discrimination Report-
    ed · by Middle-Aged and Older Persons." Social Forces,
    Vol. 55, March, 1977, pp. 728-742.

This article was based on a sample of 398 Black, 373
Mexican American, and 373 White residents of Los Angeles County, aged 45-74, who were asked about their
experiences with race and age. Each ethnic subsample
identified both race and age discrimination as common
in the country today. Smaller percentages of each
ethnic subsample (20%-45%) reported that their own
friends and acquaintances had experienced race or age
discrimination. Finally, respectively smaller percentages of each group (8%-34%) directly identified personal experiences with race or age discrimination.
The author concludes that Blacks were considerably
more likely to assert the existence of race discrimination at each of these three levels of observation
than were Mexican Americans, who, in turn, were moderately more likely to report race discrimination at
each level than were Whites. Differences among the
ethnic subsamples were less dramatic and less consistent for reported experiences with age discrimination
at the three levels of observation, although Black respondents still tended to report greater exposure to
age discrimination than the other ethnic groups, concludes the author.

Koening, Ronald, et al. "Ideas About Illness of Elderly
    Black and White in An Urban Hospital." Aging and
    Human Development, Vol. 2, August, 1971, pp. 217-225.

The authors contend that the Blacks evidenced great
regard for the hospital where they were lodged and were

(Koening, Ronald, et al.)

satisfied with the doctors. Particularly they tended, more than Whites, to prefer the young doctors who
can be expected to have been more positively influenced by changing racial attitudes than other physicians. The writers found that in many respects both
Black and White aged patients shared common views
about illness. They were equally inclined to be real-
istic about the seriousness of the illness and did not
often attribute illness causes to fate or "God's
will." They conclude that both groups seemed to regard illness as a problem to be solved and not necessary and predictable concomitant of age.

Kosberg, Jordan I. "Differences in Proprietary Institutions Caring For Affluent and Nonaffluent Elderly."
Gerontologist, Vol. 13, No. 3, Autumn, 1973, Part 1,
pp. 299-304.

The author surmises that being old, poor, and Black
compounds the probability of placement into an inferior institution, or preclusion of placement into an
Extended Care Facility (ECF) or expensive facility
which can meet higher standards. This group of elderly are often on welfare and would be placed in institutions caring for welfare aid recipients. It was
pointed out that one-third of Blacks over 75 years of
age were receiving Old Age Assistance, while only 1
out of 20 of the Whites were. A Cook County (Ill.)
Department of Public Aid reported that in 1966 of all
Blacks in nursing homes, 82% were on Old Age Assistance. He concludes that the elderly poor, who are
mainly Blacks, are often institutionalized in small,
old, and substandard nursing homes; most converted
from private dwellings. The elderly Blacks are further inconvenienced by being placed in facilities
which are located further from their families and previous dwellings than is true for the affluent elderly
who are usually White. The poor Black elderly are
also treated differently by professional and non-pro-
fessional staff members.

McCaslin, Rosemary, et al. "Social Indicators in Black
and White: Some Ethnic Considerations in Delivery of
Service To The Elderly." Journal of Gerontology,
Vol. 31, January, 1975, pp. 60-66.

A random sample of elderly clients utilizing the In-
formation and Referral Service of the Houston Areawide
Model Project were interviewed, using DHEW's Social
Indicators for the Aged. An analysis of that data by
ethnic group revealed that Anglos scored lower than
Blacks in all areas measured and that scores of

(McCaslin, Rosemary, et al.)

Blacks in this client group were essentially the same
as those of Blacks in the general population, while
scores of Anglos in the client group were consistently
lower than those of Anglos in the general population.
The findings of this study have led the authors to two
conclusions: (1) services to the aged, such as those
of the Houston Areawide Project, will be utilized by
a larger proportion of Black elderly than Anglo elderly due to more widespread need among the Black population; (2) at the same time, services will be under-
utilized relative to the needs of the Anglo population
due to a greater reluctance to admit need for services.

McPherson, Judith R., et al. "Stature Change With Aging
   in Black Americans." Journal of Gerontology, Vol. 33,
   January, 1978, pp. 20-25.

Five hundred Black Americans were measured to determine if there was a statistically significant decline
in height with increasing age. The following conclusions were found. (1) The Black population has a
greater decrease in height with aging than does the
White population. (2) Black males decrease approximately 4.2 cm in height every 20 years compared to 1.2
cm in the White population. (3) Black males below age
60 have a longer arm-span than Black males over 60.
(4) Black females decrease in height approximately 3.4
cm per 20 years. (5) Incidence of skeletal disease
is more noticeable in Black females than in Black males
and also increases with aging. (6) Black females
weigh more than Black males except in the "older" age
group.

Messer, Mark. "Race Differences in Selected Attitudinal
   Dimensions of the Elderly." Gerontologist, Vol. 8,
   Winter, 1968, pp. 245-249.

This article indicates that race differences among the
elderly account for considerably more of the variation
on three important attitudinal dimensions than differences in age, sex, marital status, education, or
health. The importance that may be attached to this
finding is primarily due to the fact that, while the
other traits have been examined repeatedly in studies
of aging, race has been largely ignored. The writer
concludes: (1) elderly Blacks have higher morale than
elderly Whites; (2) elderly Blacks have less of a feeling of integration with overall society than elderly
Whites; (3) elderly Blacks are less likely to deny
their actual age status than elderly Whites.

Quadagno, Jill S., et al. "Maintaining Social Distance in a Racially Integrated Retirement Community." Black Aging, Vol. 3, Nos. 4 and 5, April and June, 1978, pp. 97-112.

The author concludes that it is clear from the survey data that few differences exist between Black and White residents in this retirement community. While Blacks tend to be somewhat more diversified in terms of income and education, these differences are not statistically significant. Blacks and Whites tend to participate equally in activities, both in the retirement community and outside it in the wider community. They tend to feel the same about their living situation. In spite of this similarity of background, behavior and feelings, racial tension does yet exist. This tension appeared slightly in the survey data, but was really only obvious after extensive field work, argue the authors. They point out that the expressed satisfaction of the residents seems to contradict the concern about racial issues. However, these findings are not really contradictory. Residents maintain tranquility by artificially creating a means of maintaining social distance. By defining formal structured activities as work, they are able to interact comfortably in these situations. It is only in leisure-type activities where the potential for intimate friendships exists that tensions interfere with daily interaction. The implications of these findings suggest that an increase in formal activities in integrated housing may reduce racial tension and segregated patterns of interaction, conclude the writers.

Rosen, Catherine E. "A Comparison of Black and White Rural Elderly." Black Aging, Vol. 3, No. 3, February, 1978, pp. 60-65.

This article discusses interviews that were conducted on 694 ambulatory rural elderly residing in a high poverty region. They were designated as probable members of an extremely high risk population. Interviewer-respondent's race was matched in order to reduce respondents' inhibitions. Of the respondents, 48 percent were Black and 52 percent were White. Comparing the life situations of the Black and White high risk rural elderly finds that the Blacks had significantly poorer health on every index. However, 94 percent of both groups reported having a regular doctor and there were no differences between ethnic groups on when they last saw a doctor, declares the author. There were no significant ethnic differences in home ownership, but the housing conditions of Blacks were significantly poorer than those of Whites. Only 29 percent of the sample owned cars (mostly White). There was a significant relationship between race and source of retirement in-

(Rosen, Catherine E.)

come. About half of each ethnic group was supported
completely by Social Security. Twice as many Blacks
(33%) as Whites (14%) received public assistance and
twice as many Whites (33%) as Blacks (15%) reported
other economic resources, such as pensions, savings,
or family aid. Seventy-four percent of the Whites and
48 percent of the Blacks reported their income was
enough to meet their regular needs. Trained coders'
ratings of respondents' economic resources were lower
than respondents' own ratings, states the writer. All
the rural elderly reported few social interactions,
but Whites had significantly less than the Blacks.
Blacks had significantly more social resources than
Whites. During crises, Blacks turn to their families,
social agencies, physicians, and other community help-
ers for aid, while Whites turn to their families or go
it alone. The writer suggests that there was a significant relationship between the race and/or the sex
of the elderly person and their primary needs. Females reported greater loneliness and transportation
needs. Males reported more medical problems. Blacks
reported greater financial and housing problems.
Whites reported more emotional or family problems and
concerns about entering nursing homes. More Whites
(40%) than Blacks (26%) were not receiving any kind of
social or health services. Whites were more critical
of the lack of community services for the elderly.
Morale was related to race. Blacks were either more
optimistic or more pessimistic than Whites, concludes
the author. She also argues that these findings have
implications for the service needs and service delivery to rural Black and White elderly, especially
those at the poverty level.

Rubernstein, Daniel I. "An Examination of Social Partici-
pation Found Among a National Sample of Black and
White Elderly." Aging and Human Development, Vol. 2,
August, 1971, pp. 172-188.

The writer asserts that contrary to prevailing assumptions, the Black elderly are no more alone and isolated than are the general elderly population, and their
emotional state of well-being is no different from
that of the White elderly. He concludes that the
Black elderly as well as the White elderly are grown
and matured adults who are at that stage of life,
where, in the socialization process, they socialize
others, rather than being socialized themselves. It
is therefore incumbent upon us to recognize that the
Black elderly must not be viewed as children and adolescents, concludes the author.

Sauer, William. "Morale of The Urban Aged: A Regression
Analysis By Race." Journal of Gerontology, Vol. 32,
September, 1977, pp. 600-608.

The author argues that his research, though supporting only a limited number of the hypothesized relationships, while at the same time explaining what is
to the consensus a fair amount of the variance, did
offer some support for activity theory. He concludes
for both aged Blacks and aged Whites: (1) There is a
direct relationship between the health of elderly
people and morale. There is a direct relationship between the number of solitary activities an individual
engages in and morale. In addition, for aged Whites:
(1) There is a direct relationship between the frequency of interaction with family and morale. (2)
Males are more likely to manifest high morale than females.

Thune, Jeanne M. "Racial Attitude of Older Adults." Gerontologist, Vol. 7, September, 1967, pp. 179-182.

The writer surmises the results obtained in his early
analyses of differences between older Whites and older
Blacks indicate that older Blacks are less prejudiced
than older Whites; older Blacks believe they are different from both other Blacks and Whites in that they
value personal qualities rather than material objects
or pleasure-oriented behavior; and older Blacks feel
they have less personal control over their environment and are more controlled by forces outside themselves than do older Whites. The author also found
for both older Blacks and Whites a relationship between the amount of prejudice expressed on a social
distance measure and the personal feeling of internal
vs. external source of control. She concludes those
older adults who feel more inner control are those who
indicate they would behave in a less prejudiced manner
when participating in an inter-racial social situation.

_____, et al. "Interracial Attitudes of Younger and
Older Adults in a Biracial Population." Gerontologist,
Vol. 11, Winter, 1971, pp. 305-309.

The authors declare that the interracial prejudice as
it occurs within young, middle-aged, and older Blacks
and Whites and the degree to which prejudice is affected both by episodes of civil violence and by the
passage of time have been the focus of a continuing
program of research in the Southern city of Nashville,
Tennessee. Data indicate that while age affects racial attitudes, particularly the attitudes of White
Southerners, race is an even stronger determiner of

(Thune, Jeanne B., et al.)

prejudice. There were significant differences in the
degree of prejudice expressed by Blacks and Whites of
all age groups, the magnitude of these differences increasing systematically across age groups due primarily to the higher prejudice of older Whites. The
authors conclude that Blacks of all ages stated that
they were willing to interact with Whites to a greater
extent than Whites of any age stated they were willing
to interact with Blacks.

Weinstock, Comeilda and Ruth Bennett. "Problems in Communication To Nurses Among Residents of a Racially Heterogeneous Nursing Home." Gerontologist, Vol. 8,
Summer, 1968, pp. 72-75.

The writer states that all of the Black patients re-
acted favorably to their roommates, and 75% were satisfied with their neighbors. In marked contrast, only
a third of the White patients were satisfied with
their roommates and one-quarter with their neighbors.
In general, the response of Blacks indicated enthusi-
asm while the White patients showed marked disaffec-
tion. The author states that differences in reactions
and types of communication to nurses were found among
White and Black patients in a proprietary nursing
home. Strained interaction between patients and staff
members appeared to result from negative reactions of
White patients to the Black staff. They conclude
strained interaction did not seem to be a function of
staff members' negative attitudes toward the aged
since it was reflected mainly in the attitudes of the
White group.

Wellin, Edward and Eunice Boyer. "Adjustments of Blacks
and White Elderly to The Same Adaptive Niche." Anthropological Quarterly, Vol. 52, January, 1979, pp. 39-
48.

This article discusses three public housing projects
for the elderly. The writers argue that in these projects, Black and White residents make different adjustments in terms of church membership and other formal
social participation, patterns of friendship and help,
leadership, and leisure activities. They conclude
that both daily neighborly contact and desirable organized activities seem to promote more frequent and
harmonious interracial contact than is common outside
the project. These studies were conducted in Milwau-
kee, Wisconsin.

Wershow, Harold J.   "Inadequate Census Data on Black Nurs-
     ing Home Patients." Gerontologist, Vol. 16, February,
     1976, pp. 86-87.

     In the course of the investigation on Black and White
     Nursing Home Patients (NHP), the author's findings led
     him to the conclusion that census data on Black pa-
     tients in nursing homes (NH) are grossly in error.
     The 1960 census states that there were, at the time,
     no more than 6 Black NHP in NH in Alabama that are
     "known to have nursing care" (KHNC), all in state and
     federal institutions, all males over 80 years of age.
     The author later learned, in questioning the 1970
     data to be presented herein that, even in 1960, there
     were already several Black proprietary NH in existence,
     all of whom were KHNC. Yet the census somehow missed
     all of them. The author asserts the situation has not
     improved with publication of the 1970 census. The
     author concludes his study discovered at least 197
     Black NHP, 76 males and 121 females, residing in four
     black-owned NH KHNC in Jefferson County, Alabama. All
     are certified and licensed as "skilled nursing homes"
     and "extended care facilities" by Medicare and Medi-
     caid, and licensed by the State Health Department.

28.   RESEARCH ON THE BLACK AGED

Ehrlich, Ira F.   "The Aged Black in America--The Forgotten
     Person." Journal of Negro Education, Vol. 44, No. 1,
     Winter, 1975, pp. 12-23.

     The author (1)critically reviewed the literature with
     particular emphasis on the education component; (2)
     related his empirical research and methodology for
     the training of gerontologists; and (3) recommended
     roles in the gerontological education and training
     which university and community can perform to enhance
     the quality of life for Black Aged. The writer con-
     cludes that educational institutions can and should
     meet their responsibilities to the Black aged popula-
     tion by (1) creatively developing a network of infor-
     mal educational opportunities in which he can partici-
     pate, and (2) by training professional gerontologists
     with emphasis on recruitment of more Black students
     into the field. Dr. Ehrlich declares broadening the
     living horizons of the Black aged person through these
     augmented resources can provide him with the opportun-
     ity of no longer being labeled the forgotten person.

Hill, Robert B.   "A Profile of Black Aged." Minority Aged
     in America. Institute of Gerontology, University of
     Michigan-Wayne State University, Ann Arbor, 1972,
     pp. 35-50.

     The title tells what this work is about. The author
     discusses various aspects of the Black aged such as

(Hill, Robert B.)

population, education, marital status, life expectancy, family size, housing, poverty, health, and employment. The writer points out that since 1970, the
Black aged population has been increasing more than
twice as fast as the overall Black population.

Jackson, Jacquelyne J. "The Blacklands of Gerontology."
Aging and Human Development, Vol. 2, 1971, pp. 156-
171.

Dr. Jackson discusses "The State of the Literature,"
"Health, Life Expectancy, and Race," "Social Patterns,
Policies, and Resources," "Psychology and Race," and
"Related Literature." She points out that two of the
most critical research needs are mental illness among
the Black aged, and trends in the use or non-use of
nursing homes by the Black aged. The writer concludes
that while it is no longer true that almost nothing is
known about Black aged, it is still true that we have
got a long way to go! She further states that it
would be helpful if some of the research, training,
and service needs already identified in her article and
elsewhere were executed with greater speed.

_____. "Negro Aged: Toward Needed Research in Social
Gerontology." Gerontologist, Vol. 11, Spring, 1971,
pp. 52-57.

This article has three major purposes: 1. That of
providing both a brief survey of social gerontological
literature concerned with Blacks and a selected bibliography of the most useful researches presently
available; 2. That of evaluating critically these
available researches on or about Black aged; and 3.
That of conceptualizing several of the most important
research problems or areas about aging and aged Blacks
in need of further study now and during the forthcoming decade of the 1970s.

_____. "Really, There Are Existing Alternatives To In-
stitutionalization For Aged Blacks." National Conference on Alternatives To Institutional Care For Older
Americans: Practice and Planning. Eric Pfeiffer,
Editor. Durham, N. C.: Center For The Study of Aging
and Human Development, Duke University Medical School,
1973, pp. 102-107.

Dr. Jackson argues that perhaps the most important alternative to institutionalized care for old Blacks is
that practice and planning must not concentrate so
much on those who are already old. We must begin now
to concentrate more upon those who are being born today and tomorrow and tomorrow and tomorrow. We must

(Jackson, Jacquelyne J.)

make certain that we reverse this creeping tide of racism. According to Dr. Jackson we must ensure that
young Blacks will be able to grow and develop in environments permitting them to mature and to become
both independent and interdependent beings. The author believes that many of those who are Black and institutionalized in this country today are those who
have never really been allowed a chance to grow up.
That is, they have never really become adults. There
may be some critical distinctions between non-institutionalized and institutionalized old Blacks today,
with the latter remaining children and the former, despite all the odds, somehow having become adults.
Hence, the vital alternative for us is that of maxi-
mizing conditions for adult growth and development for
Blacks. These responsible Blacks will then make their
own decisions about their need for institutionalization or alternatives to institutionalization. When
health conditions do not permit them to make such decisions directly, then their spouses, children, or
other responsible family members or friends will make
the decisions for them. Dr. Jackson concludes that we
do not need to focus attention upon developing services
for aged Blacks where aged Blacks will not be able to
exercise any choice in utilizing those services and
where Blacks will have had no meaningful role in developing and implementing such services. According to
the writer we must give attention to developing aged
and aging Blacks themselves so that they can be effective producers and consumers in the market. The
types of problems to which she alludes cannot be resolved merely by changing the race of the caretaker of
the aged. Dr. Jackson also concludes that the problem
can only be resolved by individuals themselves being
allowed to make viable choices as long as they can
with the hope being that one of the alternatives to institutionalization will not be poorer care. The author argues that those aged Blacks experiencing institutionalization will find themselves in environment relatively free from stress and highly warm and receptive
to them, for many institutions now containing aged
Blacks are, intended or not, merely designed to hasten
their deaths.

_____. "Selected Statistical Data on Aging and Aged
Blacks." Proceedings of The Research Conference on
Minority Group Aged in the South. Durham, N.C.: Center
for the Study of Aging and Human Development, Duke University Medical Center, 1972, pp. 173-184.

The author states that one of the chief objectives of
this "Research Conference on Minority Group Aged in The
South" is assessing the current status of research on

(Jackson, Jacquelyne J.)

Black aged, an invaluable objective in determining
short and long-range research priorities. Another objective is emphasizing the need for an enlarging cadre
of persons trained in gerontology or geriatrics and
sincerely interested in aging and aged Blacks. Good
research can provide a strong base for planning and
action, states Dr. Jackson. These statistical data,
culled from advance and subsequent reports of the 1970
census, provide some background data on older Blacks.
At least two caveats are in order: Some modifications
of advance 1970 census data have occurred since these
tables were prepared including a reduction in the e-
numeration of aged Blacks; and a statistical picture
of Black aged fails often to portray any single aged
Black. Statistical profiles often mask the vast heterogeneity of aged Blacks. Despite these cautions,
statistical profiles have some uses, concludes the
author.

_____. "Social Gerontology and The Negro: A Review."
Gerontology, Vol. 7, September, 1967, pp. 168-178.

The purpose of this article was to provide a collection of sociocultural and psychological references on
the Black aged and to share impressions about such
references, focusing predominantly on certain emergent
issues. The author asserts that one of the present
gaps in social gerontology is empirical research on
the Black aged; and, therefore, few data are available.
Although such existing data do show some convergence,
more often their findings diverge. Dr. Jackson concludes that few valid generalizations beyond the objective socioeconomic statuses of aged Blacks are possible at the present time.

Jenkins, Adelbert H. "The Aged Black: Some Reflections On
The Literature." Afro-American Studies, Vol. 3, December, 1972, pp. 217-221.

This article gives a review of the literature on the
Black aged. Studies have shown that some samples of
aged Blacks depart from stereotypic expectations regarding their adjustment to old age, concludes Jenkins.

Kastenbaum Robert J. "Psychological Research Concerns
Relative To Aging and Aged Blacks." Proceedings of
The Research Conference on Minority Group Aged in The
South. Jacquelyne J. Jackson, Editor. Durham, N. C.:
Center for the Study of Aging and Human Development,
Duke University Medical Center, 1972, pp. 25-47.

The author contends that psychologists should be concerned about the same things that psychologically affect the White Aged as the Black Aged. Dr. Kastenbaum

(Kastenbaum Robert J.)

points out that older Blacks do not feel sorry for
themselves. He concludes that it is a pity that a
part of the population among us calling for more Black
Studies, Black History, et al., often fails to utilize
the historical talents of its best Black historians.
Among those best Black historians are many old people
who have lived through significant events which are
often not known to the young--White or Black. They
also have often had experiences which are not known to
a larger proportion of the American population--White
or Black.

Lindsay, Inabel B. and Brin D. Hawkins. "Research Issues
    Relating To The Black Aged." Social Research and The
    Black Community: Selected Issues and Priorities.
    Lawrence E. Gary, Editor. Washington, D. C.: Insti-
    tute For Urban Affairs and Research, Howard University,
    1974, pp. 53-65.

The writers highlighted some of the major problems
from which aged Blacks suffer. They also focused on
major strengths which may be brought to bear for cor-
rective purposes. It is pointed out that it has only
been in recent years that aging has commanded the
prominent attention of researchers in a variety of
fields, and the Black aged are still very much ignored
as a unique minority of the elderly population. It is
the very uniqueness of the experience of the Black elderly in America that makes research such a critical
issue. They only touched upon a few of the problems
and concerns that confront the Black elderly and undermine their chances to grow old in dignity and comfort.
The most basic problems related to income maintenance
and housing are further reflected in poor nutrition,
poor physical and mental health, increased vulnerabil-
ity, and high mortality. Even in the area of social
relationships, which has provided a haven of hope for
the many Black aged, we still find pockets of old
Black people in "geriatric ghettos" who live out their
lives in loneliness and isolation. It is evident from
the limited data and research that is available that
much action is needed to remove the disparities that
exist in this society for aged Blacks, contend the authors. It is further evident that such action must be
preceded by relevant research, because action in the
face of ignorance has invariably done more harm than
good, they conclude.

Smith, Stanley H. "Major Concerns: A Summing Up of Geron-
    tological Research and Training." Proceedings of The
    Research Conference on Minority Group Aged in the
    South. Jacquelyne J. Jackson, Editor. Durham, N. C.:
    Center for the Study of Aging and Human Development,
    Duke University Medical Center, 1972, pp. 152-154.

(Smith, Stanley H.)

The author states that there is an increasing urgency
for the collection of hard data on the Black Aged.
Complete reliance cannot be placed on longitudinal
studies. The time could be reduced considerably by
combining the longitudinal and the cross sectional approaches. Increasing reliance could also be placed on
smaller samples without negatively affecting reliability and validity. It may not be inconceivable to deal
with sample sizes of twenty-five by sample selection
devices based on rapidly defined social categories,
states the author. This will permit more in-depth
interviews and more precise recordings of behavioral
observations, argues the writer. Research must be
careful not to superimpose definitions of social phenomena on their subjects. This has been done much too
frequently on Black people. On the contrary, greater
emphasis should be placed on how these persons define
or conceptualize the social phenomena in question.
For example, instead of assuming that persons are not
married because they have not been "churched," one
should be more concerned with how these persons define
their relationship with each other and if they have
accepted responsibility for the functions of child
bearing and child rearing. The author concludes that
in research and particularly on Black people, it is
safe to make the assumption that there is a certain
order and, therefore, concentrate on recognizing, and
as a consequence, analyzing the nature of that order.
This might conceivably make more relevant and appropriate the methodological approach followed. Different definitions and assumptions will determine a different methodological approach. This in turn will affect conclusions and hopefully, policy, continues the
writer.

Solomon, Barbara.   "Better Planning Through Research."
     Comprehensive Service Delivery Systems For The Minor-
     ity Aged. E. Percil Stanford, Editor.   San Diego,
     Calif.: Center on Aging, School of Social Work, San
     Diego State University, 1977, pp. 19-29.

     The author argues that research should be an integral
     part of planning services including services to minor-
     ity elderly. Since research is eventually a set of
     tools, the important issue is the nature of the ques-
     tions which research is asked to answer. There are
     questions in regard to minority elderly which need
     answers, states the writer: Should there be cultural-
     ly specific programs? If so, how should they differ
     in regard to structure, content and process? To what
     extent do minority-specific variables enter into pro-
     gram evaluation? Systematic, programmatic research
     would appear to be one of the most effective ways to

(Solomon, Barbara)

arrive at answers. At the same time, the suggestion
that there is possibly not enough uniqueness about
the Black elderly to warrant special attention in research institutes is reflective of the negative valuation placed on minorities in our racist society,
states Solomon. According to the writer there are
thousands of research institutes in this country with
some very esoteric as well as mundane interests, e.g.
there is an Institute for Research in Acting; an Institute for Research in Practical Partisan Politics;
an Institute for the Study of the Future; and an Institute for the Study of Earth and Man. To suggest
that minority elderly are not sufficiently unique to
study separately in a special institute is strangely
contrary to the values and practices in the research
establishment, but entirely consistent with the low
valuation placed on our minority populations, concludes Dr. Solomon.

7.

BLACK
OLD FOLKS' HOMES:
1860–1980

Home For Aged Colored Women
Boston, Mass.
Founded ca. 1860

Home for Aged and Infirm Colored Persons
Philadelphia, Pa.
Founded by Stephen Smith in 1864 and is still in existence 1980

Home for Aged Men
Springfield, Mass.
Founded by Primus Mason for all races ca. 1868

The Colored Old Folks' and Orphans' Home
Mobile, Ala.
Established in 1871

Old Folks' and Orphans' Home
Memphis, Tenn.
Founded ca. 1880

The Liner's Harvest Home
New Orleans, La.
Established by Edward Liner in 1886

Widows' and Orphans' Home
Jackson, Miss.
Started date unknown; probably between 1880-1900

Carter's Old Folks' Home
Atlanta, Ga.
Establishment date unknown; probably between 1880-1900

St. James Old Folks' Home
Louisville, Ky.
Organized in 1887

Bethel Old Folks' Home
Baltimore, Md.
Founded ca. 1890

Crawford's Old Folks' Home
Cincinnati, Ohio
Founded ca. 1890

The Centenary Church Home
Charleston, S. C.
Organized ca. 1890

Old Folks' and Orphans' Home
Birmingham, Ala.
Started ca. 1890

Lincoln Old Folks' and Orphans' Home
Springfield, Ill.
Founding date unknown; probably between 1890-1903

Old Folks' Home
St. Louis, Mo.
Establishment date unknown; probably between 1890-
1905

Old Folks' Home
Augusta, Ga.
Establishment date unknown; probably between 1890-
1905

Masonic Home
Columbus, Ga.
Establishment date unknown; probably between 1890-
1905

Cleveland Home for Aged Colored People
Cleveland, Ohio
Started by Mrs. Eliza Bryant in 1893

Old Folks' and Orphans' Home
Kansas City, Mo.
Founded by Samuel Eason, a Black man, in 1894

Old Folks' Homes
Norfolk, Va.
Started in 1894 and was still in operation in the
late 1930's.

Colored Aged Home Association
Newark, New Jersey
Started in 1895. (Moved to Irvington, N. J. in 1905.)

Aged Men's and Women's Home
Baltimore, Md.
Started ca. 1895

Old Folks' Home
St. Louis, Mo.
Establishment date unknown; probably between 1895-
1904

Home for Aged and Infirm Colored People
Chicago, Ill.
Started by Mrs. Gabriella Smith ca. 1896 and was
still operating in 1920 on West Garfield Boulevard

Ashley River Asylum
Charleston, S. C.
Started ca. 1896

Lincoln Old Folks' and Orphans' Home
Springfield, Ill.
Establishment date unknown; probably ca. 1896

Old Ladies' and Orphans' Home
Memphis, Tenn.
Started ca. 1896

The Sarah Ann White Home for Aged and Inform Colored
Persons
Wilmington, Delaware
Founded in 1896

The Widow's Faith Home for Colored Destitutes
New Orleans, La.
Organized ca. 1896

New Bedford Home for the Aged
New Bedford, Mass.
Established in 1897 by Miss Elizabeth C. Carter

Tents' Old Folks' Home
Hampton, Va.
Organized in 1897 by a Society of Women called
"Tents." This home was still operating in the
early 1940's.

The Stoddard Baptist Home
Washington, D. C.
Established ca. 1897 by Mrs. Maria Stoddard

Home for Aged Colored Men and Women
Philadelphia, Pa.
Started ca. 1898

Old Folks' Home
Columbus, Ohio
Establishment date unknown; probably ca. 1898

Woman's Home Mission Society Home
Baton Rouge, La.
Started ca. 1898

The Negro Baptist Old Folks' Home
Richmond, Va.
Established ca. 1899 and still in existence in the
early 1940's

Green Memorial Home for the Aged and Infirm
Evansville, Ind.
Establishment date unknown; probably ca. 1899

City Home
Petersburg, Va.
Started before 1900 and was still in existence in the
early 1940's

Alpha Home Association
Indianapolis, Ind.
Founded ca. 1900

Home for Aged Colored Women
Cincinnati, Ohio
Established ca. 1900

Home for Aged and Infirm Colored Women
Pittsburgh, Pa.
Founded ca. 1900

Home for Negro Aged Men
New York, N. Y.
Founded before 1900 and was still in existence in
1943

Home for Negro Aged Women
New York, N. Y.
Established before 1900 and was still operating in
1943

Home for Destitute Children and Aged Persons
San Antonio, Texas
Founding date unknown; probably ca. 1900

Iowa Home for Aged and Orphans
Des Moines, Iowa
Founded ca. 1900

Old Folks' Home
Birmingham, Ala.
Started ca. 1900

Old Folks' Home
Chicago, Ill.
Founded by John Johnson and his family ca. 1900

Old Folks' Home
Providence, R. I.
Starting date unknown; probably ca. 1900

Rescue Home for Orphans and Old Folks
Jacksonville, Fla.
Started ca. 1900

The Lafon's Old Folks' Home
New Orleans, La.
Established by Thomy Lafon ca. 1900

Old Folks' Home
Westham, Va.
Organized by the True Reformers ca. 1900

The Lincoln Hospital and Home
New York, N. Y.
Founded ca. 1900

The Women's Twentieth Century Club
New Haven, Conn.
Organized in 1900 by Mrs. J. W. Stewart

Old Folks' Home
Richmond, Va.
Founded ca. 1900 and still operating in the late
1930's

M. W. Gibbs Colored Old Ladies' Home
Little Rock, Ark.
Established ca. 1900

Taborian Home for Aged and Indigent Members
Topeka, Kan.
Establishment date unknown; probably between 1900–
1905

Home for the Aged
Brooklyn, New York
Organized ca. 1901

Home for Aged and Incurable
Atlantic City, New Jersey
Started ca. 1901 by Dr. C. Fayerman

Old Folks' Home for Colored
Portsmouth, Va.
Started ca. 1901 and still in operation in the late
1930's

The Priscilla Brown Mercy Home
Selma, Ala.
Organized in 1902 by the City of Selma

Tent Sisters' Old Folks' Home
Raleigh, N. C.
Established ca. 1904

Colored Masonic Home and Orphanage
Linglestown, Pa.
Organized ca. 1905 by the Grand Lodge of Colored Free
and Accepted Masons of Pennsylvania

Colored Aged Home Association
Irvington, New Jersey
Established in 1905

Phillis Wheatley Home
Detroit, Mich.
Started in 1907 by the Labor of Love Circle

Old Folks' Home
Gloucester, Va.
Started in 1907

Old Folks' Home
Alexandria, Va.
Started ca. 1907

Evergreen Old Folks' Home
Savannah, Ga.
Organized in 1908

Home for Colored Aged Women
Anniston, Ala.
Started ca. 1908

Old Folks' Home
Natchez, Miss.
Founded ca. 1910 by the Faithful Few Circle of the
King's Daughters

Old Folks' Home
Pensacola, Fla.
Started ca. 1911

8.

SELECTED PERIODICALS
WITH ARTICLES
PERTAINING TO
THE BLACK AGED

Afro-American Studies

Aging

American Historical Review

American Journal of Medicine

American Journal of Orthopsychiatry

Annals of the American Academy of Political and Social Science

Anthropological Quarterly

Black Aging

Black Enterprise

Black Scholar

Cancer

Cancer Research

Crisis

Diseases of the Nervous Systems

Ebony

Encore

Family Coordinator

Freedomways

Geriatrics

Gerontologist

Harvest Years

Industrial Gerontology

International Journal of Aging and Human Development

Jet

Journal of Afro-American Issues

Journal of Black Health Perspectives

Journal of Chronic Diseases

Journal of Gerontology

Journal of Minority Aging

Journal of Negro Education

Journal of Negro History

Journal of Social and Behavioral Sciences

Journal of the American Geriatrics Society

Journal of the National Medical Association

Monthly Labor Review

Negro Digest

Newsweek

North Carolina Journal of Mental Health

Phylon

Postgraduate Medicine

Share

Social Casework

Social Forces

Social Policy

Social Security Bulletin

Strokes

Index